Your Genealogy Affects Your Health

Your Genealogy Affects Your Health

◆

Know Your Family Tree

F. Clarke Fraser, PhD, MD

Professor Emeritus, McGill University, Montreal, Canada

iUniverse, Inc.
New York Lincoln Shanghai

Your Genealogy Affects Your Health
Know Your Family Tree

iUniverse books may be ordered through booksellers or by contacting:

iUniverse
2021 Pine Lake Road, Suite 100
Lincoln, NE 68512
www.iuniverse.com
1-800-Authors (1-800-288-4677)

The information, ideas and suggestions in this book are not intended as a substitute for professional medical advice. Before following any suggestions contained in this book, you should first consult your personal physician.

Neither the author nor the publisher shall be liable or responsible for any loss or damage allegedly arising as a consequence of your use or application of any information or suggestions in this book.

ISBN-13: 978-0-595-39686-3 (pbk)
ISBN-13: 978-0-595-84092-2 (ebk)
ISBN-10: 0-595-39686-0 (pbk)
ISBN-10: 0-595-84092-2 (ebk)

Printed in the United States of America

Lovingly dedicated to Marilyn

Contents

Acknowledgments

Cover design by kind permission of Marilyn Preus, of "Silk Journey". It is a silk quilt, created by Marilyn, after a frieze by Gustaf Klimt.

I wish to thank Dr. Doreen Evenden and my son, Noel, for their careful reading and critique of the manuscript.

Preface

Most people are interested in their family trees for social reasons—whether their ancestors trace back to somebody famous (the Frasers trace back to Charlemagne, I am told), or skeletons in the family closet waiting to be discovered. But the family tree can be interesting for other reasons too. Family resemblances, for instance—how certain facial features or behaviors run in families, and what diseases. In the last few years there has been a vast increase in knowledge of human genetics, which is greatly enlarging our understanding of what and how things run in families. People are beginning to pay more attention to the things that occur in particular families and what they mean to particular family members.

If someone in your family has a certain disorder, it is useful to know whether this puts you at risk for the same disorder, whether it can be tested for, and what can be done to prevent or treat it. For example, if you are predisposed to breast cancer, you may want to seek more stringent screening. If you are predisposed to early coronary disease, it is (even more) advisable to avoid smoking, reduce weight, and get more exercise. That is why your family history can be important to your health.

To help you evaluate your family history, this book will summarize what is known about the inheritance of normal human characteristics, and of the common familial diseases. Only the common ones, because there are thousands of genetic diseases that are so rare that most people have never heard of them. Details of these can be found in catalogs such as OMIM (Online Mendelian Inheritance in Man). For our purposes, common means common enough to be familiar, as well as familial.

Advances in genetics have also widened the horizons for genealogists. The genes on the Y chromosome (which determines maleness) are transmitted only by men, and only to their sons. This means that the male half of the family tree can be tracked in the DNA. If you are related to Charlemagne through males only, a geneticist could probably prove it. There are also genes called mitochondrial genes that are only transmitted by mothers to their children. There are already companies that will track your ancestries this way—for a price.

Chapter one of this book will present you with the least you need to know about genetics to understand the rest of the book. Chapter two reviews what is known about the genetics of normal characteristics. These conditions are interesting, even though their presence in the family does not influence your health. Chapter three will deal with the common physical (as opposed to mental) disorders, and what it means to you if they occur in your family. Chapter four will do the same for behavioral characteristics, ranging from personality to the psychoses.

Review your family tree, look up the conditions you find in it, and consider whether they may be relevant to your health. You may not find all that many disorders in your family, but you are sure to find some. In my family there are close relatives with Alzheimer disease, type 1 diabetes, longevity, and stroke. And you will find lots of conditions that run in your family in chapter 2 on normal traits.

1

Genetics in a Nutshell

In 1940, when I started graduate school, genes were hypothetical. We had no idea what genes were made of or how they worked. In the past 66 years there has been a remarkable growth in knowledge of genetics. Now we know that genes are made of DNA. We know the precise structure of the DNA, and how it determines our characteristics. Through the extraordinary achievements of the Human Genome Project we now know the entire molecular sequence of the human DNA—some thirty billion bits of information. This has resulted in an enormous growth in genetic knowledge that has changed the face of medicine. Genetic screening and diagnosis are now important parts of the medical practice, and—I would never have dreamed it sixty-five years ago—medical genetics has become a recognized medical specialty.

Here is the essence of what genes are and how they work.

The Scene

First a little biogeography, a capsule summary of what genes are and how they work. Our bodies consist of trillions of cells of many different types—liver cells, kidney cells, nerve cells, muscle cells, blood cells, and so on. Each cell has a nucleus, a bag containing the thread-like chromosomes (twenty-three pairs in people), which contain the genetic material, the DNA (deoxyribonucleic acid). Each chromosome is a long strand of DNA on a protein framework. The DNA, the famous double helix, is like a rope ladder; the steps in the ladder are made up of pairs of the nucleotide bases guanine and cytosine (GC) and adenine and thymine (AT). Various sequences of these base pairs spell out the information that determines the cell's proteins, the main constituents of our bodies.

The proteins are long chains of amino acids. There are twenty different kinds, each with its own shape, electrical charges, and other properties. The proteins fit into each other, and into the membranes, like pieces of a three-dimensional jig-

1

saw puzzle. They have many functions. Some are structural proteins, such as collagen (tendons, bones), hemoglobin (red blood cells), myoglobin (muscle), and keratin (hair and nails). Some act as enzymes which catalyze biochemical reactions. Some act as receptors, specially shaped to recognize a molecular signal, such as a hormone, and transmit its message to some other part of the cell. The way the amino acids are strung together gives the protein its unique shape and function, and—here is the essence of it—the sequence of amino acids in the protein is determined by the sequence of base pairs in the DNA.

DNA—the Double Helix

The DNA is twisted into a spiral, like a rope ladder. The ropes are sugar-phosphate chains. The rungs are made of pairs of nucleotide bases, GC and AT, one base from each rope. The bases can only fit if the Gs on one rope pair with Cs on the other, and the As with Ts in a complementary relationship. Thus,

rope	SPSPSPSPSPSPSPSPSPSPSPSPSPSPSP--------
rung	CAT GTA GAA TGC GGG CTT CTT--------
rung	GTA CAT CTT ACG CCC GAA GAA--------
rope	SPSPSPSPSPSPSPSPSPSPSPSPSPSPSP--------

This provides a neat way for the DNA to replicate itself, which it must do when the cell divides. The two strands separate, and each builds a new strand, complementary to itself, the result being two copies of the original double strand. Various arrangements of the four bases also provide enough variety to make a code—the genetic code—that translates the sequence of base pairs in the DNA to the sequence of amino acids in the protein.

The Gene

For every protein there is, somewhere on a chromosome, a stretch of DNA that is its gene. The sequence of amino acids in the protein is determined by the sequence of base pairs in that stretch of DNA. Specifically, a particular sequence of three DNA base pairs (a triplet) in the gene codes for an amino acid in its protein. CAT codes for valine, GTA for histidine, GAA for leucine, and so on. For example, the left end of the gene for the hemoglobin molecule consists of a string of DNA triplets, as illustrated in the diagram, and the protein consists of a corresponding string of amino acids. Thus

(A)

```
gene      CAT GTA GAA TGC GGG CTT CTT --- --- --- ---
protein   VAL HIS LEU THR PRO GLU GLU * * * *
                                   (VAL)
```

When a mutation (a sudden alteration in the DNA structure) changes one base pair in a gene, that mutation changes a corresponding amino acid in its protein, which may change the protein's function and lead to a disease. For example, in the hemoglobin molecule (see diagram above) a mutation that changes a T in the 6th triplet to an A changes the 6th amino acid in the protein from GLU to VAL. This changes the properties of the hemoglobin protein, and causes a disease, sickle cell anemia. See "Single gene disorders" below.

The Genome

The DNA of the complete set of twenty-three chromosomes—some thirty billion base pairs—is the genome.

The Basis of Mendelian Genetics

Keep in mind that everyone receives one set of twenty-three chromosomes from each parent, so there are twenty-three pairs—46XX in females and 46XY in males. Every parent gives one member of each pair to each child. That is the basis of Mendelian genetics and the Mendelian laws which state the probabilities that these conditions will occur in various family situations.

Things can go wrong with either the genes or the chromosomes, and so there are various ways that genetic problems can cause genetic diseases.

Types of Genetic Disease

Diseases can run in families for many reasons, both genetic and environmental.

There are three main ways that genes can cause disease, and thus three types of genetic diseases: the single gene, or Mendelian, diseases; the multifactorial diseases; and the chromosomal disorders.

Single Gene (Mendelian) Disorders

As we have seen, mutations in a gene coding for a particular protein may alter the function of the protein and cause a disease such as sickle cell disease, Huntington disease, or hemophilia. These diseases, resulting from a single gene difference, are almost all rare. They follow the Mendelian laws of inheritance, so one can make precise predictions about the chance that a particular relative would also be affected. Although each one is rare, there are a lot of them; altogether, they affect about one percent of people. If the gene's base sequence is known, the mutant gene can be diagnosed by DNA analysis either before or after birth. Since Mendelian disorders are rare, they are beyond the scope of this book. If one of them occurs in your family, you may want to see a genetic counselor.

Multifactorial, or Complex Diseases

Multifactorial disorders are called multifactorial because they are caused by the interaction of many factors—at least several genes, each of small effect, interacting with environmental factors. They are the common familial diseases, such as diabetes, asthma, schizophrenia, colon cancer, and heart disease. Their genetics is complex. For each of them, there may be a dozen or so susceptibility genes. A person gets the disease if he or she inherits enough of these genes and is sufficiently exposed to the predisposing environmental factors, for example lack of exercise for coronary disease, or smoking for lung cancer. Having a near relative with one of these disorders increases your chance of getting it too, but, unlike the Mendelian disorders, not in a predictable way.

To figure out how much genes and environment contribute to a particular disease, geneticists use family studies, twin studies, and adoption studies. Family studies test whether a condition is more frequent in relatives of a person with it than in other people. If it is not, the condition is not likely to be genetic. Twin studies test whether, in twins where one twin has the condition it is more frequent in the co-twin in identical (monozygotic) pairs—which come from the splitting of one egg—than in fraternal (dizygotic) pairs—which come from two eggs fertilized at once. If it is more frequent, the condition is likely to be influenced by genes. Adoption studies test whether children resemble their biological parents, with respect to the condition, more than their adoptive parents—further evidence of a genetic influence.

Because each susceptibility gene has a small effect, they are hard to find; and even if any one of them could be corrected it would not help much. Removing the environmental factors is a much better approach.

Chromosomal Disorders

Our genome is a long string of DNA in twenty-three pieces, the chromosomes. Each human cell has two sets of twenty-three chromosomes, one set from each parent. These can be examined under the microscope, and each one identified.

Sometimes, usually due to a mistake when the chromosomes are dividing to form an egg or sperm, a child will be born with an extra chromosome, such as trisomy 21, (Down syndrome). Or a chromosome may be missing, as in XO Turner syndrome. Or there may be just a piece of a chromosome that is extra or missing. These abnormalities can be detected by microscopic examination.

The extra or missing genetic information causes developmental confusion, which leads to malformations, and often mental retardation, in a characteristic array or syndrome. The exact nature of the array depends on which piece of chromosome there is too much or too little of. These are the chromosomal syndromes, such as Down syndrome. For more on the more common ones, see chapter three under Chromosome Disorders. About 1% of children are born with chromosomal disorders, and far more appear in miscarriages and stillbirths.

Extra or missing chromosomes usually result from a mistake when the chromosomes are dividing, in the cells that will form eggs or sperm, so they rarely occur more than once in the family. The rare types that do recur would be detected by examination of the patient's and parents' chromosomes, and appropriate genetic counseling would be offered.

Drawing Your Family Tree

The main purpose of this book is to inform people about the significance of finding someone in the family with a familial disease. A good way to start is to draw a picture of your family tree. Geneticists and genealogists do it somewhat differently. The geneticist's way makes it easier to see the relationships, and to keep track of the interesting things that genealogists tend to ignore, like what people died of and what familial diseases they had. The following pedigree of my family (with some skeletons omitted) shows you how to do it.

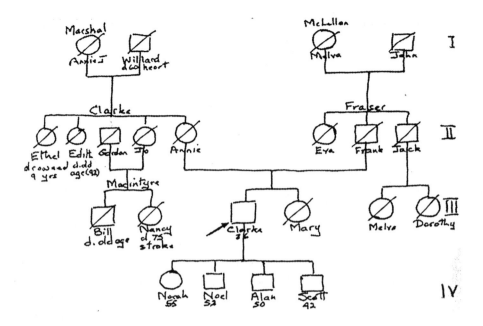

II4 Josephine. d.70, stroke
II5 Annie. d. 88, stroke
II7 Frank. d. 75, stroke
III3 Clarke. prostate ca., 68. Radiotherapy
III4 Mary. d. 37, Alzheimer disease
IV4 Noel. Diabetes type 1, onset 19

You can draw your own pedigree in the same way.

1. Start with yourself. If you are a female, draw a circle. If you are a male, draw a square. (Remember, males are squares).
2. Draw in your sibs (brothers and sisters), from left to right, in order of birth. Space them far enough apart to leave room for their children below. Connect them with a sibship line, overhead, with lines dropping down to the symbols. Write in their names, and ages, if living. Draw a diagonal line through any who have died. Draw in their spouses (or at least mates) connected by a horizontal marriage (mating) line underneath, where appropriate.
3. Draw in your mother and her sibs, in their order of birth, on the line above. Again, leave enough space for their children.
4. Draw in your father, likewise. Connect your parents with a marriage (mating) line, underneath, and drop a line to your sibship line.

5. Draw in the children of your parents' sibs—your first cousins, in the same way.
6. Draw in your mother's parents and your father's parents.

This is about as far as you need to go, as far as diseases are concerned. Diseases in more distant relatives are so far removed, genetically, that they will not alter your risk significantly. Of course if you find the same disease in more than one relative, you may want to trace it farther back, to see if it shows a Mendelian pattern.

You can number the generations, as I did, and number the individuals in each generation for easier referral, if you like. Leave some space below the pedigree, to record diseases of particular persons, and other details of interest.

It is sometimes useful to name specific groups of relatives. Your parents and children are your first-degree relatives; your uncles, aunts, grandchildren, and grandparents are second degree; and your first cousins and great-grandparents are third degree. It goes by the number of steps separating them from you. A child of your first cousin would be your first cousin once removed, a fourth-degree relative.

Finding the Genes

In the following chapters there will be references to genes being mapped, and genes being identified. Here is a brief explanation of what this means.

Finding a gene usually occurs in three stages.
1. If a disease, call it P, appears to run in families, pedigrees can be analyzed to see if it follows the laws that Mendel first worked out in the pea for single gene differences. If it does, then there must be a particular gene for P. But where in the genome is it?
2. Thanks to the Human Genome Project, we know the sequence of DNA base pairs for the whole human genome. Scattered throughout the genome are thousands of genetic markers, harmless DNA differences of which the exact place on a particular chromosome is known. These can be differences in "neutral" (not harmful) genes, or even in single bases (see SNPs in the glossary). They can be used to map P. If P is close to a marker, they will stay together within the family. If P and the marker are far apart, they tend to get separated when the chromosomes are shuffled as they go from parent to child. So family studies are done to see if P runs in families with a particular marker (see linkage in the glossary). If it does, then the gene for P must be in the same chromosome region as the marker. That is, the gene for P has been mapped to a particular chromosome site.

3. But where in the site? The next step is to search the base pair sequence of that region of the chromosome for a sequence in which one base pair is different in people who have P from those who do not. If so, that base pair must be in the gene for P. The gene for P has been identified in molecular terms.

Identifying human genes has been helped by the fact that the mouse has many genes with similar structure and function. It is often easier to identify a gene in the mouse, where crosses can be controlled after which the same base sequence can be searched for in the human.

Knowing the molecular basis for the P gene is useful; P can be diagnosed by a DNA test. Knowing what the gene does provides better understanding of the disease, and an opportunity to design better drugs for it.

Most of the conditions covered in the following chapters are multifactorial; they are not caused by major genes, but by several genes of small effect, interacting with environmental factors. These are much harder to find than the major genes. But new approaches are being developed, and some progress is being made.

DNA Enriches Genealogies

Until recently, genealogists had to rely on historical records to construct family trees. The recent advances in DNA technology have added a new tool to their armamentarium—mitochondrial DNA and Y-chromosome DNA.

Mitochondrial DNA (mDNA)

Not all of a person's DNA is in the chromosomes. Mitochondria, packages of enzymes in the cell cytoplasm that convert nutrients into energy, have their own DNA (mDNA). Since mitochondria are transmitted to the next generation through the egg, and not the sperm, all children get their mDNA from their mother. The mDNA, like the chromosomal DNA, has variability in its base pair sequences. This provides a way to trace ancestry through the female line, which is being used more and more for identification.

Y-Chromosome DNA

The Y chromosome determines maleness and is transmitted only from father to son. Tracing markers on the Y chromosome is therefore a good way to trace male lineages.

DNA Used to Trace Families

DNA analysis is used for forensic purposes—disputed paternity, and criminal and disaster victim identification in particular. But there are also uses that enlarge the scope of genealogy by adding a biological means to the historical ways of tracing the family history. Here are a few examples.

-Is it true that my great-grandmother was a Native American/Filipino/West African?

Many DNA markers are more frequent in some ethnic groups than others, so if you have an ancestor from another ethnic group, you are likely to have an increased frequency of markers from that group. Using these ethnic differences, it is possible to separate humans into four major ethnic groups: Native Americans, who migrated from Asia to inhabit South and North America; Indo-Europeans—Europeans, Middle Easterners, and South Asians from the Indian subcontinent; East Asians—Japanese, Chinese, Koreans, Southeast Asians, and Pacific Islanders; and Africans, who came from sub-Saharan Africa, the ancestral home of all humans.

It is now possible to check these markers in a person's DNA and estimate what proportion of that person's ancestors came from each of the four groups. Of course, that will not tell you which ancestors came from which group, but it's a start.

-Are those bones really those of the Romanovs?

In 1918, Nicholas II, the former czar of Russia, his wife, and five children were shot and buried by the Bolsheviks. Eighty years later, mitochondrial DNA was extracted from the exhumed remains, and compared with that of several maternal descendants, including Prince Philip of England. The samples matched, showing that the bones really were those of the Romanovs. But there was no match for the DNA of Anna Anderson, who claimed to be descended from Nicholas' daughter Anastasia.

-Did Thomas Jefferson really have a child with a slave girl?

Jefferson was accused by a disgruntled reporter of fathering a child, Thomas Woodson, by a slave, Sally Hemings. DNA analysis provided a way to check out this rumor almost two hundred years later. Thomas Jefferson did not have any sons, but his paternal uncle did, and he must have had the same Y chromosome as Thomas. Several descendants (through the male line) of Thomas Woodson did not have this Y, so Woodson was not fathered by Thomas Jefferson in spite of perhaps being named after him. But the male descendants of Eston, Sally's youngest son, did have the Jefferson Y, so Thomas Jefferson could have been Eston's father. But so could a number of his relatives, including his brother Randolph who lived in the vicinity. DNA analysis will provide some answers but not all of them.

-Is there a lost tribe of Israel in South Africa?
The book of Exodus tells that when Moses led the Israelites out of Egypt, God decreed that Moses' brother Aaron and his male descendants would be their high priests, the *kohanim*. Today many Jewish priests have the name Cohen or variants thereof. If this were true, many of the *kohanim* should have inherited Aaron's Y chromosome. Sure enough, DNA analysis has shown that about half of the priests have a characteristic pattern of markers on the Y chromosome—the Cohen haplotype—that was quite rare (5%) in other Jews. It looks as if Aaron's Y is still around more than a hundred generations later.

Furthermore, it has traveled extensively. For instance, there is a south-African, Bantu-speaking tribe, the Lemba, who have a legend that their ancestors were Jewish and came by boat from the north, perhaps Yemen. They practice circumcision and have some Jewish taboos (for example, the eating of pork). In the Lemba population, about two-thirds of the Y chromosomes have a Middle Eastern pattern, and many have the Cohen haplotype. So the folk lore was confirmed. Some of Aaron's male descendants must have wandered as far afield as Africa, and left his Y chromosome there!

If you wonder if that family with the same surname is related to you, or are curious about something in your ancestry, there are companies who (for a price) will analyze your Y chromosome, mitochondrial and ordinary DNA and perhaps provide some answers. To find some companies, just Google "DNA and genealogy."

2

Family Resemblances: Common Normal Traits

By common traits, I mean those that you are likely to have heard of, with frequencies of, say, one in five hundred or more births. Most common normal traits do not show simple Mendelian inheritance. Normal traits, such as ear shape or musical ability, are likely to be complex, so their inheritance will be complex. I list here some of those, if a) they are interesting, and b) something is known of their genetics. I admit that, since most normal traits are multifactorial and the genetics of normal traits is not of much interest to most geneticists in this molecular age, some of the findings below are not as solid as one might wish, but that's all there is.

Since the conditions I have chosen do not fit neatly into categories, I have listed them alphabetically.

Absolute Pitch

Absolute pitch (AP), also called perfect pitch, refers to the ability to recall specific musical pitches without a reference pitch. A person who has it can tell you "that phone is burbling at E above middle C." It has a frequency of around 10 or 15% in music students, and is increased by early musical training. In a recent US study, the frequency of AP in the sibs of music students with AP was 16%; in the sibs of those without AP, it was only 1%. The results suggest a genetic predisposition with an important environmental influence. The frequency is higher in Asians than Caucasians. AP is not correlated with musical pitch recognition (see below).

Asparagus Urine

Many years ago, I used to try to amuse my class by telling them how it had been shown that some people who eat asparagus produce urine that smells of asparagus, whereas others do not, and urging them to check it out. The trait was said to occur only in the presence of two mutant genes, one from each parent (recessive inheritance). Many years later, it was claimed that this was not so. The difference was that some people (about 10%) can smell asparagus in the urine of people who have eaten it and others cannot. This sharp difference (whichever it is) is likely to be genetic, but which difference is it? Do some people excrete the asparagus smell and others do not? Or do some people smell the asparagus smell and others do not? Maybe both? See also Ability to Smell Asparagus under Sense of Smell. Here is a chance for you to make a contribution to genetic knowledge. Tell me what you find in your friends and relatives, and I will put it in the next edition.

Athleticism

The basis for athletic excellence is so complex that to sort out its genetic basis would be an overwhelming task. Yet a beginning is being made.

For example, what is it about Kenyans that produces the best long distance runners? Why does West African ancestry produce the best sprinters? No environmental or cultural factors have been identified. Kenyan runners have longer, slimmer limbs, so it takes less energy for them to swing their legs. They also have more effective lactate metabolism—better for long distances. West African athletes are taller, heavier, and have muscles with more fibers (type II) that hold lots of sugar and the enzymes that burn it for the fast energy needed for sprints.

The search is on for underlying genetic differences, and some are being found. For instance, one form of a gene for a protein that binds actin (a contractile protein) to skeletal muscle is frequent in elite sprint athletes, and the other form is more common in endurance athletes. But genetic engineering to create Olympic medalists—already referred to as gene doping in the literature—is a fantasy.

Baldness

Hair loss in older age is presumably multifactorial, and sex-influenced, since it occurs much more often in men, though I do not know of any good data. Pattern baldness (starting at the forehead and receding) with onset before about thirty years of age is, according to the conventional view, one of the few common traits that seems to fit Mendelian expectations. The postulated gene, not on the X-chromosome, causes baldness when present in one dose in males, but not in females, and only occasionally in females with two doses. It seems that the pattern bald gene works only in the presence of androgen, the male hormone. It has not been mapped.

But as usual, things are not that simple. Recent studies have shown that a mutation in the androgen receptor gene, on the X chromosome, may account for about half the cases.

Blood Groups

The blood groups are important because blood transfusion should be done only between people of compatible blood groups, and because some blood group differences between mothers and their unborn babies put the baby at risk for a severe anemia (hemolytic disease of the newborn).

Blood groups reflect antigenic differences in molecules on the surface of the red blood cells. An antigen is any molecule the body recognizes as foreign and builds a defense against. It may do this by making an antibody, which will combine specifically with the antigen to neutralize its harmful effects. This immunological reaction sometimes has adverse side effects. For example, when red blood cells are exposed to an antibody against the antigen on their surface, they clump together and break down (hemolysis) with unpleasant consequences. This is what happens in a transfusion reaction, and in Rh disease (see below).

ABO Blood Group System
The most important blood group system in the blood transfusion field is the ABO system. The ABO gene, on chromosome 9q, exists in three forms: A, B, and O. Of course any one person can carry only two of them. Both the A and B genes produce an antigen; the O gene does not. So a person with two Os is group O, a person with an A and an O is group A, and so is a person with two As. And similarly for B. In Caucasian populations, most people are group O (46%) or A (42%); 9% are B (though higher in Mongolia), and AB is the rarest (3%).

In the ABO system, unlike the other blood groups, there are naturally occurring antibodies to the A and B antigens. A person's blood serum contains antibodies to whatever A and B antigens are not present on their red cells. Group O individuals have both anti-A and anti-B antibodies in their serum. Group AB persons have neither. Group A persons have anti-B antibodies, and group B persons have anti-A antibodies. If, for instance, a group B person is transfused with A or AB blood, the anti-A antibody in the recipient's serum will combine with the A antigen on the donor red cells, which then clump together (agglutination) and break down (hemolysis)—a transfusion reaction. Any transfusion where the recipient serum has antibodies against an antigen on the donor cells will be incompatible. That is the reason why bloods are cross-matched before transfusion. Can you figure out why group O persons are known as universal donors and group AB persons as universal recipients?

Rh/CDE System

The Rh system, so called because the antigen was first found in Rhesus monkeys, has three closely linked genes, C, D, and E, with their alternative forms, c, d, and e. Antigen D is the one that causes most trouble with incompatibility. The d form does not produce an antigen. About 15% of Caucasians have two of the d gene (dd), so they lack antigen D and are D-negative. The rest are Dd or DD and are D-positive.

If a D-negative person is transfused with D-positive blood, they may develop anti-D antibodies, so that if another D-positive transfusion is given, a transfusion reaction may occur. This may happen between a mother and her baby. If a dd (D-negative) mother has a D-positive baby, some of the baby's red cells may leak back through the placenta during the birth process and cause the mother to produce anti-D antibodies. If a subsequent baby is also D positive, the anti-D antibodies from the mother may pass to the baby and cause the baby's D-positive red cells to break down—a condition known as hemolytic disease of the newborn, Rh disease, or erythroblastosis fetalis—which can cause brain damage, deafness, and death. The baby is given an exchange transfusion to wash out the antibodies. This reaction used to occur in about 1 in 200 births. But now, dd mothers who give birth to D-positive babies are given RhoGAM, an anti-D gamma globulin that clumps the baby's D-positive cells and prevents the immunization. Rh disease has virtually disappeared in the developed world. This is an outstanding example of the use of genetic knowledge in preventive medicine.

Forensic Use of Blood Groups

There are many other blood groups, such as MNSs, P, Lutheran, Kell, Lewis, Duffy, Kidd, and the X-linked Xg. Most of them do not cause transfusion problems or erythroblastosis fetalis. Beside their interest to population geneticists, they may be useful in establishing (or rather ruling out) identity in cases of disputed paternity, or crime suspects.

If blood left by a criminal at the scene of a crime is of a different blood group than that of the suspect, that is evidence of innocence. If the blood groups are the same, it is not proof of guilt—other people have the same types—but the more blood group systems that are alike, the higher the probability that the suspect is the criminal. In the most famous case, that of O.J. Simpson, DNA markers were used rather than blood groups. DNA markers, being more numerous and variable, have largely supplanted blood groups for forensic purposes.

Blood groups were also used in cases of disputed paternity; if the baby had a blood group that could not have come from the mother or the putative father—say the father was AB and the baby O—the real father must have been someone else. But if both father and baby are group O, the putative father could be the father, but so could a lot of other men. Again, the more blood group systems are genetically compatible, the more likely it is that the putative father really is the father.

When Charlie Chaplin was accused of being the father of a certain child, blood group tests showed that he could not have been the father. But the court, on the basis of compassion rather than evidence, ruled in favor of the mother. In court, sympathy may trump science.

Body Odor

Very little is known about the genetics of human body odor—you can imagine how difficult it would be to do a study—but each person has an individual scent, as any bloodhound will tell you, and twin studies suggest that this has a genetic basis.

In mice, which are easier to work with, body odor is influenced by the HLA genes of the immune system. There is some evidence that this may be so in people too. Women found that men with the most pleasing body odors were those whose HLA genes were most different from theirs. So genetics can even get into your love life.

For a clear-cut example of a gene influencing body odor, see Ear Wax.

Color Blindness

The main color-blind genes are on the X chromosome—of which females have two and males only one—and also a mostly inert Y chromosome. A single dose of the color-blind gene causes color blindness in males, who have no second X to cover it; females need two doses. That is why color blindness occurs mostly in males and is transmitted to them by their (usually) normal-vision mothers.

X-linked color blindness, or more precisely, red–green color vision defect, affects about 8% of Caucasian males, and very few females. These males, as you might have guessed, have trouble distinguishing reds from greens. One of the earliest descriptions of the condition was by the English scientist John Dalton of atomic theory fame. In 1798, he clearly described the X-linked pattern of inherit-ance—transmission from males to males by unaffected females—although he did not know about genes and Mendel's laws.

The condition is more of an annoyance than a serious problem in modern soci-ety. Color-blind men have to learn how to read stoplights, and may miss some of the flags in PowerPoint presentations, and they may not be welcome in certain occupations. On the other hand, color blindness may be an advantage in some circumstances. Color-blind men were used in World War II to spot camouflage from the air—they were not deceived by the distracting color variations. This advantage could explain why the condition is so frequent; color-blind hunters may have been better at tracking the trails of game through the forest, resulting in selection for the gene.

There are two common types of severe color blindness: 1% of males have defec-tive red perception (protanopia) and 5% have defective green perception (deuter-anopia). There are corresponding milder defects: protanomaly (1%) and deuteranomaly (1.5%) varying greatly in their severity.

Thanks to DNA technology, the molecular basis of color vision and its defects is well known. I will spell out the biology, albeit briefly, to show how molecular analysis has elucidated the genetics.

The retina has two types of light-sensitive cells—rods and cones. The cones regis-ter color by means of a photopigment that absorbs one type of light—blue, green, or red. There are three corresponding types of cone cells, each containing one type of photopigment. Red–green color blindness results from mutations in the genes controlling the red and green pigments, leading to changes in their absorption spectra. Defects in blue pigment perception are very rare.

Molecular analysis shows an unusual arrangement of the genes. The red and green pigment genes are quite similar and are lined up in tandem. The normal X chromosome has one copy of the red pigment gene and one or more (up to five) green pigment genes. This means that when the chromosomes pair before forming the sperm or egg and exchange material (crossing over), they may align unevenly because the two sorts of genes are so similar. This occasionally results in unequal crossing over leading either to duplications or deletions in the red–green complex, or fusion genes—red at one end and green at the other. If some of the red gene is deleted, defective red perception results; the severity depends on how much is missing. Deletions in the adjacent green gene lead to defective green perception. Again, the severity depends on how much is missing. This explains the great variability in type and severity observed.

Dalton would probably have been intrigued to learn that DNA analysis showed that he was a deuteranope.

It is interesting that among males with normal color vision, differences in the red pigment gene cause differences in perception of red light. In other words, some men see red differently than other men. So which is the real color? The color of an object can be measured objectively—by the wavelength of the light it reflects—but its perception depends on how the light is absorbed by the red photopigment in the retina. Color is literally in the eye of the beholder.

On the practical level, if you are a male and have problems distinguishing colors, you may have a genetic color vision defect. There are simple tests that can specify which type you have. This can be useful in helping you recognize and deal with your color discrimination problems and choose lifestyles that minimize them. Contact lenses may help. Color vision may be worse at night, but night vision may be better.

If you are a male with a color vision defect, look for it in your brothers and mother's brothers but not your children (unless your wife is a carrier), since it is very probably X-linked. And don't argue with your wife about hues in that picture or quilt—or anything else for that matter.

Consanguinity: Risks for Offspring

Marrying a close relative has been taboo in some societies, particularly Judeo-Christian ones, from time immemorial. Laws prohibiting marriage between relatives vary widely from state to state in the United States and from country to country. There are also religious prohibitions. In Canada, for example, the Anglican Church forbids first-cousin marriages and the Roman Catholic Church requires a dispensation. Many U.S. states ban first-cousin marriages by law, and in some it is criminal.

On the other hand, in some Asian and African societies consanguineous marriages are favored, as they may confer some benefits, such as legal and property rights, and the stronger position of the woman when she has relatives in her husband's family. The Egyptian pharaohs took it to the extreme, practicing brother-sister mating, and seem to have gotten away with it. Even in Western societies, there are many examples of distinguished people—Charles Darwin, for example—who married their cousins without any disastrous results—quite the contrary, in fact.

Why the disapproval of marriage between relatives? Does it have any genetic basis? The short answer is that there is a small increase in the risk of the children having a genetic disorder. Some of the risk comes from recessive genes, which are harmless in one dose but cause trouble when inherited from both parents. An unrelated couple are unlikely to carry a mutant gene for the same recessive disorder. If the couple are related, they have two grandparents in common, so the chance that they both inherit the same recessive gene from one of them is much greater.

How much of a risk is there for the children of related couples? Family studies suggest that children of first-cousin parents have about a one in one hundred chance of inheriting a severe, recessively-inherited disorder. This is far greater than the chance for unrelated parents (about one in one thousand), but it would be viewed, at least by optimists, as fairly small. The increase in risk for children of second cousins is so small that it is difficult to measure. Children of first-cousin marriages also have a small increase in risk for multifactorial traits. The risk of having a child with a severe malformation (cleft lip, spina bifida and anencephaly, heart malformations, etc.) is about doubled, from around 2% to around 4%.

Of course if someone in the consanguineous couple's family has a recessively-inherited condition, the risk may be significantly increased, depending on the person's position in the family; a genetic counselor could figure out how much.

The statistical risk must be taken in its social context. I was once consulted, independently, by the fathers of two cousins who had fallen in love (the cousins, not the fathers) and wanted to get married. I saw the two fathers separately and provided exactly the same facts, objectively, to each. One of the fathers reported back to the family that Dr. Fraser had said the risk was very low and that there was no objection to the marriage. The other father said that Dr. Fraser had stated that cousin marriage could lead to all sorts of horrible problems and was to be avoided. Yet they both had the same facts!

It is hard to get reliable data on the results of incestuous mating (father-daughter, brother-sister), but what evidence there is suggests a high frequency (perhaps up to 50%) of stillbirth, severe malformations, and mental retardation.

Neither are there good data on uncle-niece and aunt-nephew matings. The risks appear to be somewhat higher than those of first-cousin matings, but much lower than those for incestuous matings.

In summary, the children of first cousins don't seem to run as big a risk as generally thought. The small increase in risk of severe disorders should be weighed against the positive things the mating might contribute—social advantages and the good genetic qualities the couple may contribute. Genetic counseling can provide figures for the particular family situation.

Thanks to advances in DNA testing, cousins contemplating marriage can now be screened for an increasing number of deleterious recessive genes and offered prenatal diagnosis.

Ear Lobes, Attached

In most people, the ear lobe extends below the point where it attaches to the head, but in some people the lobe merges with the skin of the face, making it hard to wear earrings. Some claim that the attached lobe is recessively inherited, but there are intermediate types, so it may be more complicated than that.

Ear Pits

Pinhead-sized depressions in the skin just in front of the upper attachment of the ear, or on the rim of the ear, occur as a normal variant in about 1% of people, and somewhat more frequently in African Americans. They sometimes show dominant inheritance—caused by a mutant gene in a single dose. If they occur with deafness, cysts in the neck, or other anomalies, they may signal a syndrome; genetic counseling would be indicated.

Ear Wax

Almost all Caucasians and African Americans have brown, wet, sticky ear wax (cerumen). In Asians and Native Americans the common type is grey, dry, and flaky. Intermediate frequencies of the two types occur in populations of Eastern Europe, the Middle East, the Pacific Islands, and South Africa. The gene for the wet type is dominant—caused by a gene in a single dose. It has been mapped to chromosome 16.

This may not seem all that exciting, but its interest quotient rose when the same gene was associated with body odor. In the secretory glands that produce the wax, there are globules of fluid that contribute to the wax. In people with wet wax there are many globules; in those with dry wax they are rare. There are similar glands in the arm pit that make substances that are broken down by bacteria, and are the source of body odor. In people with dry wax these glands are much smaller than in those with wet wax, which is presumably why whites and African-Americans tend to be smellier than Asians and Native Americans. When the first white men reached Japan, they were called *bata kusai*, butter stinkers, because their unpleasant smell was attributed to their eating butter. But really it was in their genes!

Eye Color, Hair Color, and Skin Color

These three topics are considered together, as they are obviously highly correlated.

First, a little biology. The pigments that color the eye, hair, and skin are eumelanin, giving a brown to black color, and pheomelanin, a red pigment. Melanin is carried in pigmented particles called melanosomes, which are carried in pigment-bearing cells called melanocytes. The color of the iris, hair, and skin depends upon the size of the melanosomes and their shape, concentration, and distribution. The enzyme tyrosinase is involved in the synthesis of melanin. (A mutation in the tyrosinase gene can lead to loss of tyrosinase activity so, in the absence of the normal gene, no melanin is produced. This is the cause of one type of recessive albinism.)

Eye Color

Conventionally, eye color refers to the color of the iris. It is often stated that blue eyes is recessive to brown eyes. Probably no other trait has been used more often as an example of recessive inheritance. But you have only to look into the eyes of your friends and relations (at least if you are Caucasian) to conclude that it cannot be that simple. And thank goodness. Wouldn't it be boring if there were only blue and brown eyes?

I became aware of this misconception early in my teaching career when I pointed out that, by the Mendelian rules, two blue-eyed parents could not have a brown-eyed child. After the lecture, a brown-eyed young man came up and said, "But sir, both my parents have blue eyes." I stopped using that example.

The irises of identical twins are so similar that the color variations must be highly heritable. There are so many gradations of eye color and variations in pattern that the inheritance must be complex. True blue eyes have little, if any, melanin in the front part of the iris. Darker eyes have correspondingly more melanin. The structure of the iris also influences its color.

In general, genes for the darker eye colors tend to be dominant to those for the lighter colors; that is about as far as one can go. Several eye color genes have now been mapped which may help to clarify the situation. Don't forget that the color of a baby's eyes may be much lighter than it will be in later life.

Hair Color

As with eye color, the genetics of hair color is complex. There is also a considerable amount of environmental interaction, particularly in the environment of the beauty salon. The genes for darker hair colors tend to be dominant to those for blonde hair. Several genes have been mapped.

It was previously thought that red-haired people carried two copies of a red hair gene, one from each parent (recessive), only visible in blonde-haired people. But it is more complicated than that. Molecular genetics is beginning to sort it out. Much of the variation comes from the receptor for the melanocyte stimulating hormone, called MC1R. The melanocyte stimulating hormone (MSH) regulates the proportion of eumelanin (black pigment) and pheomelanin (red pigment), and the MC1R gene regulates the MSH gene. People with certain forms of the gene for MCIR have a predominance of pheomelanin in their hair and skin, which is presumably why red-haired people tan poorly and are at risk from ultraviolet radiation, e.g., for skin cancer. These genes also increase the probability of having freckles. More than sixty-five forms of the human MC1R gene are now known, so the inheritance is expectably complex. It is too early to have figures for the various types.

Skin Color
Racial differences, and the fact that identical twins are much more similar than dizygotic pairs in skin color, show that skin color has a strong genetic basis. Since there is a continuous range of skin color shades from black to fair, and obvious sources of environmental variation, the inheritance must be multifactorial. The dark skin of the black races, in Africa probably evolved as a protection against the damaging sunlight of tropical climes. As our early human ancestors migrated into northern climes, the lighter skin presumably evolved to give our skins a better chance to produce vitamin D in the less available sunlight.

As for eye and hair color, the genes for the darker skin colors tend to predominate over those for light colors. Molecular genetic analysis is beginning to sort out some of the genetic factors—see, for instance, the entry for Hair Color.

Skin color is probably the trait most often used in defining "races," but very little is known of the underlying genetic differences. One thing that does seem to be clear is that the old-wives' tales about a fair-skinned couple with African ancestry having black babies have no substance. I have tried to trace a number of such tales told to support racist arguments. In every case, it was impossible to document the claims. A good rule of thumb is that if one parent is fair skinned, the child will not be much, if at all, darker than the other parent.

Hair Color—see Eye Color

Hair Form

The form of the hair—straight or curly—depends on its cross-sectional shape, which is circular in straight hair and elliptical in curly hair. Some have proposed that there is a single gene for hair form with two forms of the gene, straight and wavy. If you have two of the straight form, your hair is straight. If you have one straight and one wavy form, your hair is wavy. And if you have two of the wavy form, your hair is curly. But it can hardly be as simple as that as there are so many degrees of curliness.

There is a rare dominant gene that causes kinky hair in Caucasians. It is not clear whether the kinky hair of West African peoples involves the same gene. Data from the Human Genome Project may provide answers. The straight hair of Asians is said to show dominant inheritance, but there are not many data.

Hair Whorls

On the back of the head, where the bald spot usually occurs, about 90% of people have (or had) a hair whorl that goes clockwise; in 10% it goes counterclockwise. This difference seems to be under the control of the same genes that determine handedness. People with at least one "right" gene have a clockwise whorl. In people with two "neutral" genes, half have a clockwise and half have a counterclockwise whorl. Thus, left-handers have an increased frequency of counterclockwise whorls (about 45%). That handedness and hair whorl direction are both indications of embryonic asymmetry, and are controlled by the same genes, suggests that the process by which the embryo decides that its two sides are different is under genetic control.

That homosexuals also have an increased frequency of counterclockwise whorls (about 30%) suggests that a predisposition to homosexuality is established early in prenatal development, at least in some individuals.

Hand Clasping

When you fold your hands, which thumb is on top? Do you always do it the same way? Probably. This is a sharply determined characteristic, with about 55% of Caucasians preferring the left hand to be uppermost and 44% the right. Only 1% have no preference. One would expect such a clear-cut difference to have a simple pattern of inheritance, but it doesn't. There are racial differences in frequency, but only a modest, and complex, familial tendency. Hand clasping does not seem to be related to arm folding or to handedness.

Handedness

About nine of every ten people are right-handed. The rest are left-handed or ambidextrous—i.e., non-right-handed. Being left-handed is something of a nuisance, but much less so than in the past; there is much less social discrimination than there used to be. Being left-handed may even be an advantage, for instance in sports involving dual confrontations such as boxing, fencing, tennis, and baseball.

Left-handedness certainly runs in families, and family, adoption, and twin studies all suggest a combination of genetic and environmental factors. If you have a left-handed parent or sib, your chance of being left-handed is about doubled—i.e., about 20%. If both your parents are left-handed, your chance is about 50%.

There is a plausible theory that fits the facts quite well. It supposes that there is a gene for "rightness," and a form of the gene that is neutral. People who have two of the neutral form go either right or left at random. The search is on for such a gene.

As for environmental factors, apart from social pressures, it is curious that left-handers (and, intriguingly, schizophrenics and children with neural tube defects) are more likely to be conceived in May or June and less likely to be conceived in November or December. An ingenious hypothesis relates this to the photoperiod, the periodic variation in sunlight exposure with maximal exposure in June, and minimal in December. The increased sunlight increases certain toxic molecules in the mother's blood that could damage the embryo's brain at a stage when the embryo is deciding which side is which, and interfere with this decision. Also, left-handed mothers have more left-handed offspring than left-handed fathers do, suggesting some factor in the uterine environment.

The frequency of left-handedness appears to be increased in patients with a variety of disorders, including schizophrenia, autoimmune diseases, asthma, migraine, autism, and cleft lip. No one knows why. These associations are significant statistically, but for the individual they are not very significant. If being left-handed doubles your risk of becoming schizophrenic from 1% to 2%, will that be a worry?

It is interesting that the same genes that influence handedness also seem to influence the direction of the hair whorl on the back of your head. Most people (90%) have a clockwise hair whorl, but left-handers have an increased frequency of counterclockwise whorls (see Hair Whorls).

These findings suggest that genes are involved in determining how the body decides that its two sides are different. The early embryo is symmetrical, both sides being the same, but soon becomes asymmetrical as the heart goes to the left, the two sides of the brain become different, and so on. The process of acquiring asymmetry is, indeed, under genetic control; left-handedness (and a counter-clockwise hair whorl—see above) can be considered as a failure of this process. As the brain asymmetry involves language, identifying the genes involved in handed-ness may help in understanding human neurological development and evolution; the geneticists are just beginning the search.

Homosexual men also have an increased frequency of left-handedness, and of counterclockwise hair whorls (about 30%), which suggests a genetic predisposi-tion for at least some cases of homosexuality.

Height—see Stature

Hitchhiker's Thumb

When (if) you hitchhike a ride, does the top half of your thumb bend back more than thirty degrees? About one in four Caucasians say yes. This is said to be a recessive trait. That means that if your parents don't have it, and you do, each of your sibs has one chance in four of having it too. Check it out in your friends and relations.

Homosexuality

Homosexuality appears to run in families but not in a simple fashion. There are some who claim that the genetics of homosexuality is not even a fit subject for study. Nevertheless, there have been some studies, which are summarized below.

In one study, 52% of the monozygotic (identical) co-twins of homosexual males were also homosexual, as were 22% of dizygotic (fraternal) co-twins—higher than the population frequency of about 10%. This suggests that both genes *and* environment are involved. Male homosexuals appear to have more gay brothers than gay sisters, whereas lesbians have more gay sisters than gay brothers, suggest-ing that the predisposing factors are at least partially distinct in men and women.

Quite a stir was caused by a study that looked at the families of homosexual brothers and found a pattern suggesting that there was a gene on the X-chromo-some predisposing to homosexuality. Some of the brothers' uncles and male cousins were homosexual, but only if they were related to the original pair of brothers through females, and there was no transmission from father to son, sug-gesting that the gene is on the X-chromosome. The putative gene was mapped to the tip of the long arm of the X-chromosome. A smaller study did not confirm the X-linked pattern, and the verdict must be considered moot. Further research is needed, but is anyone looking? It must be very hard to get ethical approval, or funds, for such a project. It may well be that there is a major X-linked gene that sharply increases the chance of being homosexual, which is present only in a small number of families.

That there may be such a gene in people is somewhat supported by the finding of a homosexuality gene (named fruitless) in the fruit fly, drosophila. A male fly with the fruitless gene courts other males instead of females. The protein product of the gene has been identified, but no one knows how it acts, though it may have something to do with a neurotransmitter, serotonin. It remains to be seen whether the fruitless fruit flies court males for the same reasons that human gay males do, but, no doubt, someone is searching the human genome for a DNA sequence like that in the fruitless fruit fly. Stay tuned.

One bit of evidence in favor of a genetic predisposition for at least some cases of homosexuality is that homosexuals have an increased frequency of left-handed-ness and of counterclockwise hair whorls. See Handedness for the details.

Intelligence

We all know what we mean by intelligence, but we find it hard to define. The dictionaries do not help much: "quickness of understanding and reasoning; capacity to know or understand"; "readiness of comprehension; ability to exercise the higher mental functions."

However you define it, intelligent behavior requires a brain that is properly built, and functions well. Anything that results in an ill-constructed brain, or that inter-feres with its function, will result in diminished intelligence.

Imagine an auto show. The performance of the cars depends on their design, the quality of the materials they are built from, and their skillful tuning. Performance will vary according to these factors. Some cars will perform well and others, less well-designed, constructed, or tuned, will function poorly. Dropping a wrench into any of these moving motors, or putting water into the gas, results in poor performance, no matter how well the engines are designed and built. And a poorly-designed or ill-constructed engine will not work well, no matter how good the fuel and tuning. Similarly, brains vary in the quality of their design (genetic), construction, tuning, and fuel (environment).

I am talking about intelligence in the normal range, not the conditions resulting from mutant genes and environmental traumas that spoil the function of an otherwise normal brain and result in mental retardation.

Even though almost everyone knows what is meant by intelligence, it is not so easy to measure. There have been arguments about whether there is some kind of factor for general intelligence—a "g factor," which makes a brain function better. Or are there only capabilities for specific functions: numerical reasoning, language skill, space appreciation, and so forth. There is now a lot of evidence that there is indeed a g factor, as well as factors influencing a variety of specific skills, and that both are influenced by genes.

There is also ample evidence that intelligence is influenced by the environment. Nutrition, both before and after birth, exposure to toxins such as lead, and the degree of mental stimulation provided by the baby's environment are particularly important.

The vast amount of evidence that genes strongly influence intelligence is too large to review here. Some people seem to have an almost superstitious reluctance to admit this relation, as if intelligence was so socially important that we do not like to think that it could be determined, even partly, by genes. Perhaps some of the resistance stems from the idea that the effects of genes are immutable, which they may not be. We cannot ignore the fact that the capacity of the brain to function depends on how well its components are put together and how well its cells function. In the brain, as in other organs, this depends in large part on genes. Why should intelligence, which emerges from the brain, be any different?

The genetics of intelligence has created more social furor than that of any other trait. The evidence that genes do influence intelligence comes from family studies, twin studies, and adoption studies. Estimates of heritability range from 0.4 to 0.8—that is, from 40% to 80% of the variation in intelligence is due to genes. Nevertheless, there was resistance to the idea, particularly after claims were made that social class and racial differences in intelligence are due, in part, to genes. One such claim, made in a book called "The Bell Curve," by Herrnstein and Murray, created such an outcry that a group of fifty-two respected psychologists bought a full-page ad in the Wall Street Journal (Dec 13, 1994) that "outlines conclusions regarded as mainstream among researchers on intelligence, in particular, on the nature, origins and practical consequences of individual and group differences in intelligence." I think that this is a fair and reasonable statement and will paraphrase some of its conclusions:

- Intelligence involves the ability to reason, plan, solve problems, think abstractly, comprehend complex ideas, learn quickly, and learn from experience.

- Intelligence, so defined, is measured well by intelligence tests.

- Whatever IQ tests measure, it is of great practical and social importance. A high IQ is an advantage in life because virtually all activities require some reasoning and decision making.

- Differences in intelligence certainly are not the only factor affecting performance in education, training, and highly complex jobs, but intelligence is the most important.

- Individuals differ in intelligence due to differences in both their environments and their genetic heritage.

- That IQ may be highly heritable does not mean that it is not affected by the environment. IQs do gradually stabilize during childhood, however, and generally change little thereafter.

- Although the environment is important in creating IQ differences, we do not yet know how to manipulate it to raise low IQs permanently.

It is clear that there are no genes with major effects on normal intelligence, but numerous genes with small effects. That means that "intelligence genes" will be hard to find. There is no need to worry (as some ethicists do) about prenatal diagnosis being done to select children with superior intelligence. Ethicists also seem concerned about gene therapy being used to improve genes for intelligence; that is also very unlikely to happen.

Whether there are racial differences in intelligence is a controversial question which produces more heat than light. Here is my attempt to put the voluminous literature into a nutshell.

It seems clear that the average IQ is somewhat lower (about ten points or so) in blacks than whites, and whites average lower than Asians, in spite of all attempts to allow for the effects of cultural differences. We have to admit the possibility that these differences are at least in part genetic. It should not be surprising that racial groups may differ in the frequency of genes that influence intelligence as they do for genes for other traits. No one protests a statement that blacks are, on average, better athletes than whites, and that this is probably due, at least in part, to genes. Or that the differences in average height between races are not due entirely to differences in the environment.

If we do admit the possibility of genetic, racial, and social class differences in intelligence, so what? Racial intermixing is diminishing differences between racial groups, and migration between social classes, in both directions, will oppose the social stratification of intelligence genes. We suggest that there are environmental factors that shift the IQ downwards in all racial groups, but more so in the poor, and therefore more so in blacks. This effect is far more important than that caused by any genetic differences between groups. Efforts to correct this deplorable state of affairs by improving the environment will get us a lot farther than arguing about genetic differences.

Perhaps the reason that people are upset by the idea of racial differences in intelligence is that this results in even more racial discrimination. People are inclined to reason, falsely, from the general to the particular. Because the mean of the bell curve for blacks is somewhat lower than that for whites, it does not mean that "blacks are dumber than whites" as some would have it. It tells you nothing about any particular individual from either race. You cannot infer that because a man is black his IQ is lower than his white neighbor's. A man should be judged by what he is—kind, honest, industrious, and yes, even smart—not by his religion or the color of his skin. Then racial discrimination would disappear.

On the individual level, since the genetic basis for intelligence is multifactorial, it follows that, on average, the intelligence of a child is likely to be intermediate between the parental average and the population average. But as there is a good deal of assortative mating (people tend to marry those of similar intelligence), the children will tend to be closer to the parental value than the population value. There is a good deal of spread of course. On average, sibs differ from one another by twelve IQ points. Whatever genes your children may have inherited, their intelligence will benefit by a nourishing, stimulative environment.

Longevity

Does longevity run in families? Yes, but so many things influence longevity that it is hard to sort out how much is due to genes much less identify them. There are rare major genes for conditions that shorten life span, called progerias, but none that I know of that lengthen it, at least in people.

Family and twin studies estimate the heritability of lifespan as around 25%, not very strong. Genes influencing lifespan have been identified in round worms, fruit flies, and mice, and some of these, and other genes, are beginning to be mapped in people. Ongoing genetic studies of the whole Icelandic population, and of long-lived Ashkenazi Jews may eventually find some of them. In the meantime, we can only evoke the old aphorism about choosing your parents well. Statistically, if you have a long-lived parent or sib, your chances of living a long life are almost doubled. But life spans are increasing so rapidly one may well ask "double what?"

Multiple Births—see Twinning

Musical Pitch Recognition

A study of English twins estimates the heritability of musical pitch recognition as 71%. People with poor musical pitch recognition are called "tune deaf" or "tone deaf." The trait is likely to be genetically complex. Musical pitch recognition is not to be confused with absolute pitch (see above), which is not correlated with musical pitch recognition.

Perfect Pitch—see Absolute Pitch

Premature Graying of Hair

This entry refers to premature graying in otherwise healthy people, not to the graying that occurs with the premature aging syndromes and a variety of other disorders.

I could not find any statistics on the frequency of premature graying. From personal observation I would guess that it is somewhere around 1%. There are also no good data on its inheritance. That it runs in some families as if caused by a single gene difference (dominant) is as much as can be said.

There are some studies that find premature graying associated with diminished bone density (osteopenia), but other studies disagree. The effect, if any, cannot be very big.

Sex

Biological sex is one of the few characteristics determined almost entirely by genes. Women have two X chromosomes, and give one or the other to each child. Men have one X and one Y chromosome, and give one or the other to each child. There is a gene on the Y chromosome that makes you a male. If you do not inherit this gene, you will be a female.

In spite of this simplicity, there are many misconceptions about the determination of sex. In societies where having a male child is of the greatest importance, women are divorced for having a succession of female and no male children, as if it was their fault. In defense of these women, some will state that it is the male who determines the sex of the child. Neither side is right. The sex of the child is a matter of random chance. The male squirts a few million sperm into the female; half of them carry an X chromosome and the other half a Y. It is like tossing a coin to decide which one wins the race and fertilizes the egg. The father has no more to do with it than the mother. This idea that the male determines the sex of the child is quite common. Even Dear Abby promotes it. But it is not so.

Since the determination of sex is a matter of chance, it follows that sex, although genetically determined, is not familial. That is, having had several children of one sex does not alter the odds for the sex of the next child—about one to one (actually there is a slight excess of males, about 106 to 100, for reasons that are not clear.)

It has recently become possible to diagnose the sex of a baby quite early in pregnancy by a simple blood test, which will be a boon to those who can't wait to open their Christmas presents, but raises some hackles among the ethicists. It could be used to abort fetuses of the unwanted sex—usually female—in some societies.

The test is based on the fact that some of the baby's cells leak back into the mother's blood and break down, leaving their DNA floating in the mother's blood stream. If the baby is a boy, there will be Y-chromosome DNA in the mother's blood; if the baby is a girl, there will be no Y-chromosome DNA. So DNA analysis can diagnose the baby's sex. If the baby was not of the sex that the parents wanted, they could have an abortion without saying why they wanted it.

Of course, it has been possible to diagnose sex before birth ever since prenatal diagnosis first became possible, in the early 1970's (not counting the happening in BC 0, when the angel Gabriel successfully predicted the sex of an unborn child on two occasions). In fact, sex was the first trait to be diagnosed prenatally, by study of the fetal chromosomes. But that involved sampling the fluid around the fetus (amniocentesis), which could only be done in the second trimester, around fifteen weeks, so that an abortion, if chosen, could only be done several weeks later. Guidelines for prenatal diagnosis say it should not be done on a healthy baby, and few women, in the Western world at least, would undergo the stress of amniocentesis and a late abortion just to avoid having a child of the "wrong" sex. This new technique can be used as early as five weeks, when abortion is a much simpler matter, and since sex is not a medical condition, the medical regulations do not apply—hence the ethical problems.

It is generally agreed that aborting a fetus because it is of the unwanted sex is unethical, at least in Western countries. In certain countries (India, China) where having a son is very important, there has been a significant decrease in the proportion of female babies, resulting from a combination of prenatal diagnosis for sex selection and female infanticide. In the Western world, would prospective parents be tempted to take this blood test, which is non-invasive, inexpensive, and done early in pregnancy, to achieve a child of the wanted sex? Probably not very often. The Canadian Royal Commission on New Reproductive Technologies found that, in Canada at least, there is a very small preference for boys. Preference for one sex or the other only becomes important in families who have had several children of the same sex. And very few people said they would be willing to abort a baby because it was of the "wrong" sex. It seems likely that testing of fetal DNA in mothers' blood will be used to diagnose genetic diseases, not sex—another benefit of the genetic revolution.

Recently, a new approach to sex selection has emerged. Semen can be treated with antibodies to Y-bearing sperm removing them so the semen has only X-bearing sperm, and will produce only female offspring. Or vice versa. Once the ethical issues are resolved, sex selection before fertilization will no doubt be done in people.

Skin Color—see Eye Color

Smell, Sense of

The sense of smell depends on receptors on the sensory nerve cells in the lining of the nose—the olfactory epithelium. There are many kinds of olfactory receptors

(ORs) that register specific smells, and corresponding numbers of OR genes. Each olfactory neuron expresses only a single copy of a single OR gene out of the many; how it does this is a mystery. Thus, each neuron has a single receptor that binds to a specific range of odorants. Humans have about one thousand OR genes. Fish have only one hundred. From the Human Genome Sequence over nine hundred of the OR genes have been identified.

The genetic control of the sense of smell is obviously complex. One might expect that if each odor has a specific receptor and corresponding gene, there would be hereditary differences in ability to smell many specific odors, but only a few have been identified. For example:

- About 10% of people have a heightened ability to smell asparagus. No family studies have been done, but what else could determine this sharp difference?

- Androstenone, an androgen, smells like stale urine or strong sweat to about 35% of people, has a subtle, not offensive odor to 15%, and has no smell at all to the other 50%. But among the insensitive, sensitivity can be induced in about half by systematic exposure to the compound. Again, no family studies are available.

- The odor of musk, produced by pentadecalactone, a substance used in antiperspirant, cannot be smelled by about 7% of Caucasians. Inheritance is recessive. This trait is not found in blacks.

- A recessively inherited inability to smell the strong, distinctive scent of Freesia flowers occurs in about 4 to 10% of Europeans.

- About 1% of Caucasians and 9% of blacks cannot smell the odor of isovaleric acid, a substance present in stale sweat.

So our senses do not lie to us, do they? But it is wise to keep in mind that yours may get different messages than mine from the same signals. What does androstenone really smell like?

Stature

This entry deals with normal variations in height, not dwarfism or gigantism.

Stature is often used as an example of a multifactorial trait, meaning that it is determined by many genes, each of small effect, interacting with environmental influences of course. Final height depends on many things, including the prenatal environment, the child's hormones, its nutrition, chronic infections, and the age at which fusion of the cartilages at the ends of the long bones occurs, so they can no longer lengthen. All of these are influenced by genes and by environmental factors interacting in complicated ways.

Family and twin studies estimate that about 70 to 85% of the variation in height is due to genes (heritability). There are strong parent-child and sib-sib correlations, but also some correlation between spouses, since people tend to prefer mates of similar heights (assortative mating).

Stature, like other multifactorial quantitative traits, shows regression to the mean. Parents whose average height is above the mean will have children whose average height will be shorter than that of their parents, but taller than the mean of the population. Similarly, short parents will have children who are shorter than average, but taller than they are—on average. So, if you are much shorter than you would like to be, and would like your children to be taller than you are, choose a tall mate—and vice versa if you are too tall.

Linkage studies with DNA markers are beginning to tease out genes with a big enough effect on height that they can be detected. Eventually their DNA sequences will be identified, and how they act determined. But since they will not have large effects, don't expect any dramatic breakthroughs in the way of gene therapy for being too short or too tall.

Taste, Bitter

The ability to detect the bitter taste of phenylthiocarbamide (PTC), the substance that makes cabbage taste bitter (if it does), or related chemicals that cause goiter (thyroid enlargement), shows marked variation. The drug propylthiouracil will do almost as well as PTC if you want to test yourself or your family and friends. Use one pill to make a solution. Make several dilutions from strong to weak. Dip paper towel into the solutions and let it dry. Taste test yourself and your friends.

The difference involves the -N-C-S- chemical group. The majority of people can taste weak concentrations of the compound (tasters), but about one in three Caucasians can taste only much higher concentrations (non-tasters). This striking sensory difference shows recessive inheritance of the non-taster trait—the non-taster gene has to be received from each parent. The difference is not related to taste acuity in general.

Recent data suggest that there are several (maybe five) receptors for bitter taste, one of which involves PTC taste. The frequency of tasters is higher in people who don't like cabbage, suggesting that the bitter taste of cabbage is PTC-related. No one seems to have studied the frequency of PTC-tasters among professional wine-tasters. It is amusing to think of them arguing about whether a wine is bitter. Who would be right?

Taste, Sweet

Taste buds distributed over the tongue contain receptor cells, each of which is able to detect and signal one or more taste qualities, e.g., sweet, sour, salty, and bitter.

Ongoing research is using a combination of mouse and human genetics to find a gene that influences sweet sensitivity. Crosses between mouse strains that preferred sweet drinks and those that did not were used to map a gene (Sac) to a particular region on a particular chromosome, but it was not identified. When the draft sequence of the human genome became available, a search for sequences corresponding to the mouse Sac region located a gene that encodes a protein with the qualities of a receptor, suggesting it might be the Sac gene. Going back to the same sequence in the mouse, mutations in it were found that distinguished the taster from the non-taster strains. By the time you read this, the corresponding mutations in people will probably have been found.

A recent study has found that cats cannot taste sweets since one of their taste receptor genes for sweet is inactive. This could explain why they are carnivores.

Knowing the molecular structure of the sweet-taste receptor and its binding site will help drug designers to make non-caloric sweeteners with a cleaner sweet taste and without the health problems of sugars.

It is intriguing that eating an artichoke will make water taste sweet, but only to about 60% of people. Is this a genetic difference? Here is a research project that doesn't need a lab.

Tongue Rolling

The inability to roll the tongue into a tube was said by some to be recessive to the ability to do so, but others found a low rate of concordance in identical twins suggesting that genetics may have little to do with it. Another research opportunity that does not require a lab.

Twinning

Twins have always been a subject of interest, particularly to their surprised parents, and also as mythical, historical, or literary figures. They have been important to geneticists as a way of sorting out the relative importance of genes and environmental factors.

Identical, or monozygotic (MZ), twins result from the splitting of a fertilized egg, resulting in two genetically identical individuals—Nature's way of cloning. Fraternal, or dizygotic (DZ), twins result from the fertilization of two different eggs at the same time, and are no more alike, genetically, than ordinary sibs.

In Caucasian populations, about one in every eighty-seven deliveries is a twin birth. About one-third of these are MZ, and—you guessed it—two thirds are DZ. The frequency of MZ twins is remarkably constant, about four per thousand deliveries in various populations. Virtually nothing is known of the causes of MZ twinning. It does not seem to run in families.

The frequency of DZ twins is much more variable, presumably being influenced by the hormonal factors that influence ovulation. It varies with maternal age from near zero at puberty to fifteen per thousand births at age thirty-seven and then falls to near zero again just before menopause. The frequency is low in Mongoloid races (about four per thousand), higher in Caucasians (eight per thousand), and higher still in Nigerians (sixteen per thousand or more). The frequency of twins—and of triplets and higher order multiple births—is increasing due to the use of fertility drugs that cause multiple ovulations.

The predisposition to have DZ twins is maternally inherited, although there are a few remarkable reports of paternal transmission. For a mother who has had a DZ twin, the chance of having another one is tripled—about 3% for each pregnancy. The chance of having DZ twins is also increased in the offspring of female DZ twins.

Genes that increase ovulation rates and twinning have been mapped in sheep and pigs, but no corresponding gene has been found in people yet.

Webbed Toes

Partial webbing of the second and third toes is so common that I have included it with the normal variants. In many families it shows dominant inheritance, as it does in my family, appearing in me, my father, his father, and my aunt Eva. In a few families it appears only in females. If there are accompanying malformations, and mental retardation, it could be part of a syndrome.

3

Genetics of Common Physical Disorders

Disorders can run in families for several reasons. There are environmental causes, such as scabies or unhealthy dietary habits. The genetic causes are mostly of two types: Mendelian and multifactorial.

Mendelian disorders are caused by a single mutant gene, and follow the laws of inheritance first described by Mendel. Almost all of the Mendelian diseases are so rare that most people have never heard of them. They are rare because the people who have these diseases are likely to have fewer children than those who do not, so the mutant gene is less likely than the normal gene to be passed on to the next generation. More and more Mendelian disorders are being identified at the DNA level. If someone in your family has such a disease, genetic counseling can be sought.

There are many common diseases that also run in the family. They do not fit the Mendelian pedigree patterns, yet family and twin studies suggest that they have a genetic basis. These are the multifactorial disorders, and mapping the human genome is gradually clarifying their genetics. In a nutshell, they result from the interactions of several—perhaps many—genes, each of which increases susceptibility to the disorder in question, but not very much. A person with enough of these susceptibility genes, in the wrong environment, will get the disorder. These genes are harder to identify at the DNA level than are the genes for Mendelian disorders, but progress is being made; susceptibility genes are being located for more and more of the complex disorders. A susceptibility gene for, say, schizophrenia should not be called "the gene for schizophrenia," as happens all too often in the popular press. It is just one of the many factors contributing to susceptibility.

In this chapter I will show how the genetic revolution has added to our knowledge of the genetics of some of the familial disorders that are common enough to be familiar to most readers. This information is not intended to help in the diagnosis of the diseases or with genetic counseling, though it might help you, or an involved friend or relation, decide whether to consult a genetic counselor.

As the disorders I have chosen do not fit neatly into categories, they are presented in alphabetical order.

Alzheimer Dementia (AD)

When I first became aware of this progressive dementia (loss of intellectual function), it was considered one of the pre-senile dementias (young onset, before age sixty to sixty-five or so). Then it was realized that many patients with a later onset have the same condition. It is the most common senile dementia.

Onset is insidious, with progressive loss of intellectual faculties and, particularly, memory. The diagnosis cannot be made with certainty on clinical grounds alone, and requires microscopic examination of brain tissue. The disease results from the accumulation of a protein called beta-amyloid protein, which is produced in the brain cells in abnormal amounts from a precursor called APP, amyloid protein precursor. The normal cellular function of APP is unknown. The beta-amyloid deposits cause characteristic neurofibrillary tangles and amyloid plaques, which can be seen under the microscope at autopsy or in a brain biopsy, and provide the only definitive means of diagnosis.

Late-onset AD is somewhat familial, with a multifactorial basis, including some environmental factors, such as head injury. One genetic modifier is the APOE gene on chromosome 19, which codes for a lipoprotein involved in cholesterol metabolism. There are three forms of the gene: E*4 is associated with increased risk for AD, and E*2 may have a protective effect.

Among early-onset cases of AD, a minority (perhaps about 1% of all AD cases) have a strongly familial pattern best interpreted as due to a gene that usually, but not always, causes the disease when present in a single dose (dominant with reduced penetrance). Mutations in at least three genes may cause the disease: the APP gene and the genes for presenilins 1 and 2, proteins involved in the metabolism of beta amyloid.

In a representative Dutch study, the risk at age seventy for first-degree relatives of early onset cases (less than sixty-five) was about 13%, versus about 7% for controls. The lifetime risk (to age ninety) of first-degree relatives was about 40%, compared to 14% for controls.

So if you have a parent or sib with early onset Alzheimer disease, your chances of getting it are significantly increased, More so if there is more than one early-onset relative. If you want to know how much, a genetic counselor could work it out for you.

Late-onset AD is also familial, but less so. Here are some ballpark figures from a United States study. If you have a sib with onset of AD after age sixty-nine, and unaffected parents, your chance of being affected would be about 2% by age sixty-four, 4% by seventy-four, and 8% thereafter. If your sib had an early-onset, these figures would be 6%, 10%, and 17%. If you also had an affected parent they would be 8%, 21%, and 46%.

If you have a strong family history, genetic testing to identify the mutant gene could be offered, though it would not always be successful, and the risks, even for known carriers, are not precisely known. Many families would decline the opportunity, preferring not to refine their statistical risk. When deciding whether to have genetic testing, you might like to see a genetic counselor.

Anencephaly—see Neural Tube Defects

Anorexia Nervosa—see Bulimia

Asperger Syndrome—see Autism

Asthma

Asthma is an allergic disorder in which the bronchi respond to environmental stimuli (often allergens) by inflammation and narrowing, leading to difficulty in breathing, wheezing, and coughing.

The frequency varies widely, and seems highest in Western societies; about 10% is a ballpark figure. The prevalence appears to be rising, for unclear reasons. Atmospheric pollution seems a plausible culprit. Then there is the "hygiene hypothesis"—the culprit is the eradication of many childhood infections, and a cleaner lifestyle in general. Apparently, the immune system needs to be challenged by infections in early childhood in order to develop an effective defense system later on. Don't keep your child too clean!

Family studies, twin studies, and adoption studies all support a genetic component to susceptibility, but the inheritance is complex. In one study, 17% of the children of an asthmatic parent were asthmatic, and another 8% were probable asthmatics.

An ongoing United States Collaborative Study on the Genetics of Asthma, among others, has found evidence of linkage to several chromosome regions, pointing the way to eventual identification of specific genes. One likely candidate is T-bet, a gene that regulates a gene involved in the immune response. Asthmatics have reduced amounts of T-bet in their lungs, and "knock-out" mice that lack the T-bet gene develop asthma.

See Eczema for new information about one such gene, the filaggrin gene.

Autism

Children with autism have limited or absent verbal communication, a lack of reciprocal social interaction or responsiveness, and restricted, stereotypical, and ritualized patterns of interests and behavior. They seem to be obsessed with details without seeing their meaning. A current theory is that the problem lies in poor communication between brain areas.

Autism affects as many as one in five hundred persons—more, if milder forms are counted. Twin and family studies indicate that genes play an important role in its causation. The risk for sibs is around 5%. There are reports of an increased frequency of cognitive disorders, social functioning problems, and psychopathology in near relatives. Several chromosome regions associated with susceptibility and at least three genes on the X-chromosome have been identified.

Asperger syndrome is a mild form of autism with less impairment of speech and intellect. The two disorders may appear in the same family, suggesting that their spectrums of severity overlap.

Autism affects three to four times more boys than girls, and there seems to be an association with increased head size. Claims that it can be caused by the measles-mumps-rubella vaccine appear to be unfounded; many studies have shown no connection. The reason for the recent increase in frequency remains a mystery. It is probably real, and not just due to better methods of detection.

Bedwetting (primary nocturnal enuresis)

This is a condition all too well known to many of us. It is defined as nightly bed-wetting persisting beyond the age of seven. It affects about 10% of seven-year old children, but the frequency varies widely between populations. More boys have it than girls—three to one in one study. From the age of seven, about 15% of affected children are cured per year, so few affected children have it beyond the age of sixteen.

Genetic studies of bedwetting are not popular. One of my graduate students started to study it, but came to me in tears because of the ribald response of her colleagues when she told them what she was working on. We did not pursue that topic.

A large Swedish family study reported that, in about half the families, bedwetting behaves as if transmitted by a single gene that causes the condition in about 90% of those who carry it (dominant with 90% penetrance). Several genes have been mapped, so there is genetic heterogeneity.

Here are some risk figures for the individual family. If both parents are affected about 77% of the children have it. If only one parent has it (more often the father) about 44% of the children are affected.

There is a small group of bedwetters who have been dry for at least six months and then started wetting again. These are said to have secondary nocturnal enuresis. In this group, there is often a history of psychological stress, which may be predisposing. In the primary form the accompanying psychological stress is thought to result from, rather than cause, the condition.

Bulimia Nervosa

Bulimia nervosa (BN) is a psychiatric disorder involving episodes of binge eating, self-induced vomiting, and over-concern with body weight and shape. Both bulimia and the related disorder anorexia nervosa (AN), which involves compulsive food restriction, are strongly familial, and twin studies suggest a moderate heritability. The genetics is complex, as one might expect for such a complex trait.

BN and AN are related, but not identical. Up to half of patients with AN develop BN at some time during their illness. The frequency of AN is increased in the relatives of patients with BN, and vice versa. BN may also be related, in a complex way, to obesity. Several chromosome regions have been associated with AN or BN, but no specific genes have been identified so far. A gene for brain-derived neurotrophic factor (whatever that is) has been found to be associated with AN and BN. As more genes are identified, the picture may become clearer.

Cancer

Cancer is a disorder that starts when a single cell and its descendants, keep on dividing when they ought not to. When the processes that tell cell division when to stop are lost, the cells proliferate without control—a tumor. When the tumor does not invade the surrounding tissues, it is called benign, since it is usually less dangerous than if it does. If the abnormally multiplying cells invade adjacent tissues or spread to other parts of the body (metastasis), the tumor is called malignant. The term "cancer" applies to the malignant form.

DNA analysis has shown that the loss of control of cell division that leads to cancer can happen in many ways. Cell division is a highly regulated affair, with accelerators, brakes, checkpoints, fail-safe mechanisms, and even suicide. There are over one hundred genes involved in the control of cell division and differentiation. There are also genes for enzymes that detect mistakes when the DNA is copying itself, and repair them. There are genes for proteins that monitor the status of the cell's DNA and, if it becomes too defective, cause the cell to die. A mutation in any one of these genes may cause the cell and its descendants to multiply, uncontrollably, into a cancer. Because of the fail-safe systems, it may take mutations of several genes before control is finally lost.

There are two main categories of genes involved in cancer production: oncogenes and tumor-suppressor genes. The normal forms of the oncogenes are important for regulating normal cell growth and division. The normal form may mutate and become an oncogene, which leads to uncontrolled proliferation and cancer. Examples of oncogenes are the breast cancer genes, BRCA1 and BRCA2.

The tumor-suppressor genes suppress tumor formation. Some tumor-suppressor genes do this by preventing the cell from dividing when it should not. Others do it by causing cells with too many defects in their DNA to die.

The rest of this entry will cover, briefly, the family patterns and the genes that have been identified, for the common cancers.

Genes increasing the risk of cancer in the breast, ovary, colon, prostate, and uterus have been identified. The data are still coming in, and there are still gaps in our knowledge of risks, outcomes, and treatments.

Any figures given below are rough estimates, and subject to revision. Applying them to a particular case is a complex task, best done by a genetic counselor or cancer specialist.

Breast cancer
About one in nine women will develop breast cancer, and one in seventy-five will develop ovarian cancer by the age of eighty-five. Most cases of breast cancer have a low familial tendency. About 10% come from high-risk families with breast and/or ovarian cancers, which appear to involve a major gene mutation. These have an earlier onset, and are more likely to recur, both in the patient and in her relatives.

Several environmental factors have been shown to increase the risk of breast cancer, but the increases are not large. These include not having children or having them later in life, obesity, alcohol intake, possibly diet (? hydrogenated fats), and combined hormone replacement therapy.

Two major genes have been identified: BRCA1 and BRCA2. Over one hundred mutations have been identified in each gene. Mutations in BRCA1 or BRCA2 rarely occur in the ordinary forms of breast cancer. They were found in 30-70% of the high-risk families, in various surveys, but these may have an upward bias. Since not all families link to one of these genes, there must be at least one more BRCA gene.

BRCA1, isolated in 1994, is a tumor suppressor gene involved in DNA repair. It was thought to account for about 50% of the familial cases of breast cancer, and 85% of cases from families with both breast and ovarian cancer, but these were overestimates. More recent estimates are 13-18% and 33-40%. About one in forty Ashkenazi Jews carries a mutant BRCA1 or BRCA2 gene. The frequency is less in other populations—about 1/500 to 1/800 Caucasians. The lifetime risk of breast cancer for women carrying BRCA1 or BRCA2 is estimated as somewhere between 40 and 90%, depending on the populations sampled and individual risk factors. For ovarian cancer the lifetime risk appears to be around 30%. BRCA1 carriers of either sex have a four-fold increase in risk of colon cancer. Men have a three-fold increase in risk of breast cancer, which is still quite low, of course.

BRCA2 is also involved in DNA repair. Carriers have about the same increase in risk for breast cancer as in BRCA1 and a lower risk for ovarian cancer. There is also an increased risk of breast cancer (about a 6% lifetime risk), and perhaps for prostate cancer, in men who carry the gene.

I emphasize again that the risks provided are ballpark figures. Since the genes were identified only a fairly short time ago, the figures are not all in yet.

If you have one or more relatives with early-onset breast cancer, you may be wondering about having a DNA test to see if you are a carrier. This raises a lot of questions. For one thing, even if you do have a strong family history, it may well be that you do not carry one of the identified mutations. Secondly, would you really want to know? In one study, only about 50% of high-risk women accepted testing.

If you were shown to be a carrier, what would you want to do about it? Take Tamoxifen, which is supposed to lower the risk of breast cancer but has some side effects? Remove breasts and/or ovaries? Just do regular screening? Would your chances of getting insurance be impaired? Or even of getting a job? The issues are complex, and the answers will be different for each individual. Genetic counseling will provide risks for your particular family and, hopefully, help you to reach the best decision for you.

Colorectal cancer (CRC)
The lifetime risk for colorectal cancer (CRC) is about 6%, so it is one of the most common cancers. Both environmental (e.g., diets high in fat, low in fiber) and genetic factors are involved. Several genes are known that cause CRC in a single dose (dominant) including: *adenomatous polyposis coli (APC)*. In this rare (less than one per twenty-five thousand) condition, persons carrying the gene develop thousands of polyps in the colon, at least one of which will surely become malignant. The APC gene is a tumor suppressor. Mutation results in transition from normal epithelium to adenoma (a benign tumor), and subsequent mutation in another gene causes transition from adenoma to the malignant carcinoma. Removal of the colon is preventive, but may reduce the quality of life.

Hereditary nonpolyposis colorectal cancer (HNPCC))
This cancer accounts for about 2% of colorectal cancer cases. Most, but by no means all, cases result from mutations in the MLH1 or the MSH2 gene, both of which are involved in repairing errors in DNA replication. The mutant genes have a population frequency of about 2%. When the gene is mutant, repair is impaired, so mutations accumulate at other loci, some of which may lead to malignancy. A single dose of the gene will cause colon cancer in about 80 to 85% of carriers by age seventy—higher in men than women. There may be cancers at other sites too, particularly of the uterine lining (endometrium), with a 50 to 60% lifetime risk.

OTHER CANCER GENES

P53
This gene suppresses the development of many tumor types, regulating cell division in several ways. It is called the "guardian of the genome." For example, if a cell carries too many mutations, the P53 protein, a DNA-binding protein, will induce the cell to commit suicide, "apoptosis." If the gene is mutant, the mutant-loaded cell may not die, but become malignant. P53 is mutated in about 60% of cancer cases.

Genetic engineering that increases P53 in experimental animals appears to reduce the frequency of cancers, but also reduces life span by promoting aging. Life is very complex!

Malignant melanoma
Malignant melanoma runs in the family in some cases, but it is not clear how often or in what manner. At least two genes have been identified. Sunlight is by far the most important factor.

Prostate cancer
Cancer of the prostate is one of the most common causes of cancer mortality in males, affecting about one in nine men. African Americans have the highest frequency and Asians the lowest. Twin studies support a genetic susceptibility (around 40% heritability), but it must be complex. A number of genes have been identified that bring about a modest increase in susceptibility, and some that increase aggressiveness of the tumor.

The lifetime risk for prostate cancer is about doubled by an affected first-degree relative, increased fivefold by a first- and second-degree relative, and increased almost elevenfold by three or more affected first-degree relatives, particularly if there is an early-onset case. Affected brothers increase the risk more than affected fathers. So if you have a father or one or more brothers with prostate cancer, have a rectal exam and screening (PSA) test even more regularly than if you don't. Genetic testing is not recommended yet, as it is not yet known how much each of the known genes increases susceptibility.

Cataracts

A cataract is a cloudiness of the lens in the eye that, if it is dense enough, interferes with vision. There are many types of cataract associated with single-gene differences, but they are present at birth, or in infancy, and each is rare. Age-related cataracts appear in the elderly. About one in three British people over sixty-five have one. They are often so minor that affected people often do not realize they have it. I have had one for over ten years that my ophthalmologist can see, but I cannot. There are few studies of causes, and even fewer clear-cut results.

Twin studies suggest that genes account for almost 50% of the variation (heritability), but no major genes have been identified. Suspected environmental factors include ultraviolet light (particularly B), smoking, obesity, steroid medications, diabetes, and alcohol, but none of these plays a major role. Animal experiments show that anti-oxidants such as vitamins C and E are protective, but there have been no human trials. (A proposed trial would never get by an ethics committee).

Chromosomal Disorders

Sex chromosome abnormalities—These include:
-XO, or Turner syndrome.
-XXY, or Klinefelter syndrome.
-XYY.
-XXX.
*trisomy 21—*see Down syndrome

Club Foot

Club foot (*pes equinovarus*) is a deformity in which the foot is turned downwards and tilted inwards. It affects about two of every one thousand babies, and about twice as many boys as girls. Both feet are affected in about half the cases. Some of the mild ones will straighten out by themselves, or with a little manipulation. Others may need casting or surgery.

Twin studies suggest a genetic predisposition, and one of the predisposing genes has been mapped. Finding out how it works may help to understand how club foot happens. Maternal smoking is one of the predisposing environmental factors, particularly in genetically predisposed fetuses.

If you have a child with a club foot, your next child will, on average, have about a 3% chance of having one too.

Coronary Heart Disease (CHD)

Coronary heart disease causes one-third of all deaths in the United States. Its causes are complex. There are well known environmental risk factors, such as high-fat diets, smoking, lack of exercise, obesity, high blood pressure, and emotional stress. These interact with genetic factors that alter lipid (fat) metabolism in various ways to increase the risk of a heart attack. For example, people who carry the APOE4 form of the apolipoprotein gene are at increased risk of CHD, but much more so if they smoke. An account of the many genetic factors influencing the risk of CHD is beyond the scope of this book. As an example of the benefits of the new genetics, here is an account of some beautiful (at least to a scientist) genetic studies that help to illuminate the nature of CHD. It is a nice example of how sorting out the genes involved can illustrate the complexity of a biological process and clarify it.

First a little background. Much of CHD is associated with hypercholesterolemia, too much of a fatty compound, cholesterol, in the blood. The major culprit is low-density lipoprotein (LDL), a lipoprotein that binds to cholesterol. (Lipoproteins are proteins that carry fats). High blood levels of LDL lead to coronary disease, caused by deposition of LDLs (with cholesterol) at sites of damage in artery walls, where they contribute to the potentially obstructing atherosclerotic plaques that block the artery in a coronary attack. Inflammation is also involved in the formation of plaques. This process is also influenced by genes.

LDLs are secreted from the liver as precursors called very low-density lipoproteins (VLDLs), which are broken down in muscle and fat to the LDLs. The LDLs are removed from the blood by LDL receptors (LDLRs) on the surface of liver cells. The LDL/cholesterol particles are taken into the liver cells where they are broken down. Then the cholesterol goes into the cellular cholesterol pool.

When the cholesterol concentration is too high in the liver cells, production of LDLRs by the LDLR gene is suppressed, so less LDL is taken up, the LDL/cholesterol is retained in the blood, the liver cholesterol falls, and the blood cholesterol rises—a feedback mechanism. Similarly, when the liver cholesterol is low, the LDLR gene is activated, more LDLRs are formed, LDL/cholesterol particles are taken up more rapidly, the liver cholesterol rises, and the plasma level of cholesterol falls.

The liver pool of cholesterol is influenced by many variables, including how much dietary cholesterol is absorbed from the intestine, and how much is excreted into bile. Both of these are influenced by genes.

Understanding of cholesterol metabolism was greatly advanced by the study of four mutant genes that cause heart disease. Without the identification of these genes and their mutants, the role of LDL in CHD would still be obscure.

The four mutant genes all cause coronary heart disease by making the liver LDL receptors less active, and thus raising the blood LDL levels. The most common of these is that for familial hypercholesterolemia (FH), which results from mutations in the LDLR gene that impair or prevent formation of LDLRs. The frequency of people who carry one dose of the FH gene is at least one in five hundred and even higher in Ashkenazi Jews. People with this gene have half the normal number of LDLRs, a 2.5-fold increase in plasma LDL, and a high risk of an early (sixty years old or younger) heart attack. They account for 5% of all coronary cases. The rare person with two copies has virulent coronary atherosclerosis, and often dies from heart attacks in childhood.

The other three mutant genes are rarer. One decreases binding of LDL to its receptors. Another interferes with its transport in the liver cell. A third suppresses activity of the receptor gene.

Most of the hypercholesterolemia in the population results, not from these mutant genes, but from high-fat diets interacting with other environmental factors and poorly-defined susceptibility genes, probably influencing the feedback regulation of LDLRs by cholesterol. I am happy to say that moderate quantities of red wine seem to have a beneficial effect on LDL levels.

The other good news is that there is a group of drugs called statins, that reduce the frequency of heart attacks through lowering LDL levels by blocking an enzyme in the cholesterol synthetic pathway.

The take-home message is simple. Get lots of exercise Don't smoke. Eat a sensible diet. Keep your weight down. Have your blood pressure and cholesterol checked regularly. All the more so if you have one or more first-degree relatives with early coronary disease. If your cholesterol is up, it's up to your doctor to find out why and up to you to do something about it.

Crossed Eyes—see Strabismus

Deafness—see Hearing Loss

Diabetes Mellitus

Diabetes mellitus is a disorder of sugar metabolism involving either a lack of insulin or an inability to use it. Insulin is a hormone that (among other things) regulates carbohydrate metabolism. It is produced by the pancreatic islets.

The insulin used for treatment of diabetes used to be made mostly from the pancreas of cows. This "foreign" insulin was sometimes antigenic to humans, so that patients would become allergic to it. One of the early triumphs of genetic engineering was to isolate and clone the human insulin gene, and put it into bacteria, where it was still able to produce insulin. The bacteria could then be grown in bulk and used to produce human insulin for the treatment of diabetics without the antigenic effects of cows' insulin.

There are two main types of diabetes mellitus, as well as many rare syndromes in which diabetes is one feature.

Diabetes mellitus type 1, insulin-dependent (IDDM)
IDDM results from a deficiency in insulin production by the pancreatic islets. It has a frequency of about one to three per thousand by age seventeen, but a significant number of patients are affected after the age of twenty, so it is no longer called juvenile diabetes.

Lack of insulin results in high blood sugar. Untreated patients eat a lot, drink large amounts of water, and urinate a lot. Diabetic coma may ensue if the disease is not treated. There are long-term complications that affect the eyes, kidneys, nerves, and blood vessels. The offspring of diabetic mothers are at increased risk for malformations. Good metabolic control during pregnancy reduces this risk.

The genetics of IDDM is complex. In monozygotic (identical) twin pairs in which at least one twin is affected, less than half of the co-twins are affected, suggesting that non-genetic factors play an important role in causation. An important trigger is viral infection, which may damage the pancreatic islets—my son Noel became diabetic at the age of twenty-nine after having the flu. The damaged islet cells give rise to autoantibodies (antibodies against the person's own tissues) that destroy the islets. So IDDM is an autoimmune disease.

Several genes have been identified as increasing susceptibility to IDDM. The most important is in the HLA complex which, among other things, determines the cellular antigens involved in graft rejection. Some forms of the gene are protective and others increase susceptibility.

Sibs of patients with type 1 diabetes have an average risk of 5 to 10% of also having it. For offspring the risk is about 2% in the first decade. Modifier genes alter the risk. Having the DR3 or DR4 forms of the HLA gene increases the sib risk to as much as 19%. DR3 predisposes to autoimmune disease of the islets; DR4 predisposes to formation of anti-insulin antibodies.

Screening for islet antibodies may identify affected sibs before clinical onset which would allow preventive measures, but no such measures have been found as yet. Treatment with small subcutaneous doses of insulin and other regimes were thought to be preventive, but results of trials are not promising.

Diabetes mellitus type 2, non-insulin dependent (NIDDM)
This type of diabetes is much more frequent than type 1, affecting 5% or more of adult Caucasians, and rising. In NIDDM patients the body cells are resistant to insulin. NIDDM occurs more often in obese individuals, usually after the age of forty, and can often be controlled by diet or drugs. But about a third of NIDDM patients end up having to take insulin. If untreated, it can result in damage to the heart, kidneys, nerves, and blood vessels.

NIDDM appears to be a disease of affluence. Its frequency is increasing at an alarming rate—by 50% in the United States between 1991 and 2000—and the age of onset is decreasing. Experts think that the epidemic is being driven by the epidemic of obesity (see Obesity below). This, in turn, is being fueled by the combination of an ample food supply and a sedentary lifestyle. Diabetes is beginning to increase in many developing countries as they adopt more Westernized lifestyles and diets.

There are striking racial differences in frequency. About 13% of African Americans and 10% of Hispanic Americans are diabetic. Indigenous peoples tend to be hardest hit, at least when they adopt more civilized lifestyles. Of the adult Pima Indians of Arizona, 50% have NIDDM, the highest frequency in the world.

Researchers are working hard to find why obesity causes insulin resistance. Several hormones produced by fat cells have been implicated, as well as fatty acids. NIDDM is multifactorial, and can result from various combinations of genes interacting with environmental factors. Geneticists are busy trying to pin down the genes, but progress is slow because most of these genes will have fairly small effects, so they will be hard to find. A number of loci have been mapped to a chromosome region, but not identified at the DNA level. This is too bad, as such genes would provide good targets for new anti-diabetes drugs. This is important because the simpler approach, eat less and exercise more, does not seem to be catching on.

For first-degree relatives of NIDDM Caucasian patients, the risk is about 10% for clinical diabetes and about 20% for an abnormal glucose tolerance curve, indicating susceptibility.

There is a rare gene that causes young people who carry it to get type 2 diabetes; it is therefore called MODY (for Maturity Onset Diabetes of the Young). At least three candidate genes have been implicated. Maybe these will give us some clues about the usual type of NIDDM.

Down Syndrome

Down syndrome, or trisomy 21, is the most common chromosomal syndrome. Most children with Down syndrome have a typical appearance and are easily recognized. Langdon Down, the English physician who first described the syndrome, called it mongolism because of the slanted eyes, but this unfortunate term has been dropped, thank goodness.

Down syndrome is caused by an extra chromosome 21, which causes widespread developmental confusion, resulting in a variety of malformations and mental retardation of varying degrees. Children with Down syndrome tend to be happy individuals, and are often musical. The IQs of Down syndrome patients who have not been raised in institutions shows the same correlation with their parents' IQs as does that of their unaffected sibs, but on the average, some fifty points lower. Down syndrome patients raised in institutions tend to have much lower IQs than those reared at home.

In most cases, the extra chromosome 21 results from a mistake when the chromosomes are separating to form the sperm or (more often) the egg. The chance that the same mistake will happen again in a future pregnancy is quite small. Thus, Down syndrome is a genetic condition but usually not familial.

In a few cases (about 5%), the extra chromosome 21 has become attached to another chromosome (a translocation) and gets dragged into the sperm or egg along with the unattached 21, so the resulting individual has three 21s—one of them hooked onto another chromosome. In about half of these cases, the translocation may also be present in one of the parents. If so, the risk that the same problem will happen again is quite high. So even when the diagnosis is clinically obvious, the baby's chromosomes are checked to detect the translocation cases, which require further investigation.

The chance of having a baby with Down syndrome increases with increasing maternal age. In the late twenties, the risk begins to rise from about one in one thousand, and by age thirty-five it is about one in three hundred. By age forty-five, it is about one in forty-five. Since women are now having babies at later ages, the frequency of Down syndrome is increasing.

Prenatal diagnosis can detect the extra chromosome by examining fetal cells in the amniotic fluid, obtained by inserting a needle into the amniotic cavity (amniocentesis). For details, consult your obstetrician or genetic counselor. Prenatal diagnosis is offered routinely for any woman who is pregnant at age thirty-five or over.

More recently it has been found that a fetal protein, AFP (for alpha-fetoprotein), and several hormones, such as human chorionic gonadotropin and estriol, have levels that are altered in the mother's blood when the fetus has a chromosome problem or a neural tube defect. Many prenatal programs routinely offer a "triple test," measuring the level of AFP and two (or more) hormones in the mother's blood. Either a high value or a low value for any of the tests is an indication that there is a small chance that something is wrong, and that further investigation is indicated. Abnormal values are found in about 5% of pregnancies. Further explanation is beyond the scope of this entry. If you are concerned, consult your nearest genetic counselor.

Dyslexia

Dyslexia, or reading disability, is a heterogeneous condition characterized by unexpected difficulty in learning how to read. It affects 10% or more of children. Family and twin studies indicate a multifactorial causation, involving both genetic and environmental factors. There are some striking dominant pedigrees, but they are rare. Thanks to the Human Genome Project, specific genes for susceptibility to dyslexia will be mapped and sequenced, and their functions will be identified, which will help to clarify its causes. At least three susceptibility loci have been mapped so far.

Interestingly, researchers found that the condition is more common in English and French people than in Italians. They attributed the difference to the fact that Italian has far fewer ways of spelling the speech sounds than do English and French, so there is less room to go wrong.

There are no useful estimates of the risk for relatives, since the condition is so heterogeneous. If you have dyslexia, the chance that your sibs and children will also have it are significantly increased, but no one can say by how much, yet.

Eczema, Atopic

Eczema, or atopic dermatitis, commonly begins in infancy or early childhood, as scaly, itchy, inflamed skin. It affects 10 to 20% of children in Western societies and shows a strong familial tendency. As with asthma, the frequency appears to be increasing, for reasons that are unclear. Eczema is one of three allergic (atopic) diseases; the other two are asthma and hay fever. There is a common familial tendency. Ichthyosis vulgaris, a dry, flaky skin, also seems to be involved. About 8% of children with eczema also have ichthyosis vulgaris, and about 50% of asthmatic children also have eczema.

The common factor may be the gene for filaggrin, a protein that is an important part of the epidermal barrier that keeps water in and noxious substances out of our bodies. It has recently been found that about two of every three eczematous children, particularly those who also have ichthyosis vulgaris, have mutations in the filaggrin gene. Not all carriers of these mutations have the disease, i.e., there is reduced penetrance.

Also, in about one in five hundred children with severe ichthyosis vulgaris, certain filaggrin mutations are found in a double dose. People with a single dose of such a mutation (about 10% of the population) may have a dry flaky skin. It seems that impaired skin barrier function plays a key role in the development of atopic (allergic) disease. Discovering the role of filaggrin may show the way towards a more rational treatment.

Other genes predisposing to eczema have been mapped, but not so far identified in molecular terms. As the picture becomes clearer, more accurate family statistics will emerge.

Epilepsy

In ancient days, epilepsy was called the sacred disease because people thought that epileptics were possessed by demons and had visions that were sent by the gods. Hippocrates commented that epilepsy would be considered divine only until it was understood—which is still not entirely the case.

Epilepsy results from a large number of brain cells (neurons) firing together. Seizures may appear as a momentary loss of consciousness ("absence," or *petit mal*), an unusual movement of the body, or a convulsion. Nowadays, it is more appropriate to refer to the *epilepsies* (plural), because there are many different causes. In most cases, there is no apparent cause; epileptics are considered to have "idiopathic,"/"centrencephalic,"/"primary generalized" epilepsy. They have a characteristic brain wave (EEG) pattern.

The familial nature of idiopathic epilepsy was recognized by Hippocrates, and has been substantiated by many family and twin studies. According to one fairly representative study, the EEG trait appears in about 40% of the sibs of a child with this disorder, reaching the maximum frequency between ages five and fifteen and decreasing thereafter. Of the sibs who show the EEG pattern, about 15% have at least one seizure, and 8% have recurrent seizures, compared to 2% in the general population. This genetic predisposition to have seizures in the presence of an "epileptic" EEG also appears in children with febrile seizures, and with focal epilepsy, due to local brain damage. So the family history can be important in the evaluation of prognosis and management in a child with seizures.

Glaucoma

Glaucoma is one of the most common causes of blindness. It is associated with an increase in pressure of the fluid inside the eye.

Think of the eyeball as a balloon with a camera in it. At the front of the balloon is a lens. At the back is the retina that, like the film in a camera, registers the image projected from the lens and (not like the film) sends it on to the brain. The balloon is kept inflated by an inflow of fluid from the veins and an outflow from a canal at the front of the eye. If the outflow is blocked, the pressure inside the balloon goes up, which may damage the retina and lead to loss of vision. This is glaucoma. Actually it's more complicated than that, since some people have the pathological changes without the increase in pressure, but this is not well understood.

As one would expect from such a complex system, there are many causes of glaucoma: environmental, genetic, or, usually, a combination of the two. In a few families, the cause is a major mutant gene, some of which cause the disease in a single dose (dominant) and others only when present in two doses (recessive). In these families, the glaucoma is likely to be present at birth (congenital) or come on in childhood (juvenile). Several of these genes have been identified. For the rest, multifactorial inheritance is the rule. So if you have an affected parent or sib with adult onset, your chance of getting it is somewhat increased, to perhaps 5%. If you have more than one affected relative, particularly with early onset, you might want to consider consulting a genetic counselor, but you probably won't get a simple answer. In any case, have regular checkups with your ophthalmologist so that the condition can be treated early.

Hearing Loss

The ear is a very complex organ. It converts sound waves, by various stages, into nerve impulses in the brain. Various things can interfere with this process. The ear canal can be closed, so the air waves never reach the drum that registers the wave vibrations. There are three little bones linked to each other in the middle ear that pass the vibrations along from the drum to the inner ear. These may fuse together into an immobile rod leading to conductive (otosclerotic) deafness. In the inner ear, there are tiny hairs of varying lengths that move with the vibrations and convert them into electric impulses to send to the brain, which converts them into sound. These may be defective, as in congenital sensorineural deafness, or the hairs may wither away with age, as in presbyacusis (loss of hearing with advancing age) with which all too many of us will be familiar. Or the series of nerves that convey the impulses from the ear to the temporal lobe of the brain may not be intact.

Thus it is no surprise that hundreds of genes have been identified that, in mutant form, cause hearing loss. No doubt there are many others, which affect hearing in complex ways, but have not been identified. We will discuss, only briefly, the genetic basis of the various types of deafness. If you are deaf, or have a near relative who is deaf, you may want to consult a genetic counselor. But reading this entry first may help you to ask better questions.

There are environmental causes of deafness, of course. Prenatal infection with German measles (rubella) is one that has virtually disappeared, thanks to vaccination. The worst culprit is loud noise. One wonders how much hearing loss is due to rock bands, motorcycles, jackhammers, and other auditory insults.

Age-related hearing loss (presbyacusis)

This is the type that will be familiar to most readers, and is also the one about which least is known of the genetics. It can be considered a late-onset sensorineural deafness. Because it is so common, comes on so late in life, and is so variable in severity, it is very difficult to study genetically. In fact, I do not know of any serious attempt to do so. It is assumed that presbyacusis is caused by a number of genes, with small effect, interacting with various environmental factors in complex ways. But, unfortunately, except for loud noise, we have no idea what most of those factors are.

Otosclerosis

This type of deafness results from fusion of the bones in the middle ear that transmit the sound vibrations from the eardrum to the inner ear, so it is called conductive deafness, though there may be some nerve involvement. It affects up to 1% of adults, usually appearing in the third decade, and more often occurs in females than males. Family pedigree patterns suggest a dominant gene with less than 50% penetrance—that is, less than half of those who carry the mutant gene become deaf. Linkage has been shown to three different genes, each of which can cause the condition.

Syndromic deafness

Hearing loss may be a part of many syndromes in which the deafness is associated with other traits, such as a white forelock, visual degeneration, kidney disease, or cleft palate. There are hundreds of such syndromes, all of them so rare that they will not be familiar to most readers.

Non-syndromic sensorineural deafness (NSSD)
This type of deafness involves the hair cells of the inner ear or the nerve pathways from ear to brain. Profound childhood NSSD has a frequency of about one per thousand in Caucasian populations, but the frequency of deafness is much higher if all cases severe enough to require a hearing aid are included. Cases with loss in only one ear are more likely to have an environmental cause, but there are a few genetic types that can involve only one ear.

There are families in which sensorineural deafness not due to a syndrome (NSSND) is caused by a mutant gene when present in a single dose (dominant), and a few in which the gene is on the X-chromosome. In the remainder, the cause is a recessive gene (present in two doses) in about half the families; in the other half the cause is non-genetic. Until recently, it was impossible to tell which half any particular patient fitted into. But recently, thanks to the Human Genome Project, several dozen genes have been identified as causes of NSSND. Surprisingly, a majority have been traced to a mutation in one gene, called GJB2, which codes for one of the connexins, a group of proteins that form the channels that connect cells to one another. The same mutation can cause varying degrees of deafness, from mild to profound, in different family members. The deafness is usually non-progressive, but not always.

This has been one of the more dramatic applications of DNA technology to clinical genetics. Previously, parents of a child with NSSND were counseled that the next child had either one chance in four or a very low risk of being affected, but it was impossible to say which. Since about half the cases were recessively inherited, the risk for a sib worked out to about one chance in eight. Now they can be offered a DNA test that, if positive for the mutant gene, would put them in the one-in-four class, with the possibility of prenatal diagnosis. If negative, the risk would be much lower. Genetics centers are now beginning to include DNA testing in the regular workup of children with NSSND.

The option of prenatal diagnosis (PND) to parents of a child with NSSND is a mixed blessing. Many parents would not want to have PND feeling that the condition is not serious enough to warrant terminating the pregnancy. On the other hand, some deaf parents would ask for PND with the intention of aborting the fetus if it would have normal hearing. Although there is no prohibition of abortion for social reasons, this would contravene the geneticists' guidelines that do not approve abortion of a healthy fetus for genetic reasons.

Hemochromatosis

Hemochromatosis might be called the disease that (almost) wasn't. It is a recessively-inherited disorder of iron metabolism—the mutant gene must be present in a double dose. Patients have an excessive absorption of iron consumed in the diet and cannot excrete it all, so the iron piles up in the tissues and causes damage in various organs. There may be damage to the liver (cirrhosis), pancreas (diabetes), skin (over-pigmentation), joints (arthritis), and heart (arrhythmias, failure). The gene (called HFE) has been sequenced, and two mutations have been identified that account for almost all cases. It is not yet clear exactly how the defective HFE causes the abnormal iron transport.

Whatever the reason, there is a simple treatment: blood-letting (phlebotomy). Hemoglobin contains iron, and regular bleedings, by removing hemoglobin, deplete the iron stores and diminish the organ damage. Women have a monthly (menstrual) blood loss, which is why the disease is so much less frequent in females.

The mutant genes are quite common; about one in two hundred northern Europeans have the most common one in a double dose (homozygous). A common genetic disease, easily diagnosed, and with a simple treatment, seemed a good candidate for population genetic screening to detect the disease before it causes problems. But there was a catch.

Screening of a large population showed the expected number of people carrying two HFE mutant genes (homozygotes), but very few of these had hemochromatosis. It seems that only a few homozygotes—about 1%—actually get the disease. Geneticists call this reduced penetrance—greatly reduced, in this case. If so, population screening would not be such a good idea. Lots of mutant HFE homozygotes would be identified, but very few would actually get the disease. Others have suggested that this estimate of penetrance is too low. But penetrance is clearly not high. Further work is needed.

The message is that, in the unlikely event that you have a near relative with hemochromatosis, get tested to see if you carry the mutant gene. If you are also a homozygote, your chance of getting the disease is greatly increased over that of the population, but is still quite small, perhaps as low as 1%. Have your iron levels checked regularly and, if indicated, make a monthly blood donation to the Red Cross.

Klinefelter Syndrome—see Sex Chromosome Disorders, 47 XXY

Lactose Intolerance

Milk has a special sort of sugar called lactose. It is broken down by the enzyme lactase. In many mammalian species, the gene for lactase is turned off after the baby is weaned, as lactase production is no longer needed, and becomes an unnecessary expenditure of energy. This works well in mice and most other mammals, but in people who drink milk after weaning, it can cause problems. If the enzyme is turned off, the undigested lactose may cause nausea, gas, and diarrhea after drinking milk. In most humans the enzyme is not turned off at weaning, so there is no problem. But it is turned off in some people, leading to lactose intolerance. Thus milk-drinking humans have converted a normal trait, the turning off of the lactase gene at weaning, into an abnormal one. There is evidence that the gene for lactase persistence was selected for, beginning some five to ten thousand years ago, in groups that used dairy farming.

Lactose intolerance is recessively inherited. The gene has been mapped to chromosome 2q, so there could be a diagnostic test one day, But it is simpler to take some lactase with your milk, or just don't drink any.

Language Impairment

Children with specific language impairment (SLI) have significant language deficits in the presence of adequate educational opportunity and normal nonverbal intelligence, and in the absence of other causes of language impairment (such as hearing loss or cleft palate). They have, in varying degrees, problems with articulating speech sounds, expressing themselves verbally, and understanding the speech of others. There is a relationship with dyslexia, but its nature is not well understood.

The prevalence of SLI has been estimated as 2 to 7% in English-speaking, pre-primary-school children in various studies.

The condition is strongly familial. Twin studies suggest that genes play a major role, particularly in cases involving expressive, rather than receptive skills, but that the genetic basis is complex. SLI has been linked to regions on chromosomes 16 and 19. Definition of specific genes, in molecular terms, will surely lead to a better understanding of the nature of SLI, improvements in its diagnosis and treatment, and perhaps a better understanding of the origins of speech.

Mental Retardation

There are, of course, many causes of mental retardation, including single gene disorders, too much or too little chromosomal material, and damage to the brain from environmental factors such as maternal alcoholism, and malnutrition, or lead poisoning, either before or after birth. The remainder can be considered multifactorial, resulting from interactions of numerous genetic and environmental factors with effects that are so small they have not been identified. The continuing genetic revolution will, no doubt, identify some of these. This will increase our understanding of brain development and function, and might even lead to medications that would improve mental function. It probably will not be of much help in diagnosing or screening for mental retardation, since the susceptibility genes will each have a small effect.

For a sib of a person with mental retardation that is not part of a syndrome a ballpark figure for the chance of being retarded is around 5%. But a genetic consultation is recommended, to make sure it is really non-syndromic.

Migraine

Migraine is a headache disorder that is so common that there is probably no need to describe it. It affects about 4% of children, 6% of men, and 18% of women in the Caucasian population. Estrogen is an important factor.

The most common type is migraine without aura (MO) in which the pain is one-sided and often occurs with vomiting and sensitivity to bright light and loud sound. In migraine with aura (MA), the headaches are similar, but they are preceded by attacks of focal neurological symptoms, such as flickering lights or visual distortions. We can thank Lewis Carroll's MA for the wonderful distortions in "Alice in Wonderland."

Twin studies indicate that genes and environmental factors both play an important but complex role in the causation of migraine. Compared with the general population, the first-degree relatives of persons with MO had a threefold increase of MO. First-degree relatives of persons with MA had a twofold increase of both MA and MO.

Several susceptibility genes have been mapped. As it becomes clear how they act, so will the nature of migraine.

Milk Intolerance—see Lactose Intolerance

Myopia

Myopic, or nearsighted, people have to hold what they are looking at close to them. Myopia, like other refractive errors, is a complex disorder, involving the interaction of many genetic and environmental factors. It runs in families but not in a simple fashion. Twin studies show a fairly high heritability. Near work (e.g. sewing, intensive reading) appears to be an environmental factor that increases the probability of myopia in genetically susceptible individuals. Myopia seems to be getting more frequent, for reasons that are unclear.

Several genes are known that cause high (severe) myopia, but only 2 or 3% of myopic people have high myopia. At least ten genes that increase susceptibility to ordinary myopia have been mapped. They probably interact in a multifactorial way. One such is the PAX6 gene, known to be important in eye development.

If you have a myopic first-degree relative, your chances of being myopic are increased, but I could not find any figures as to how much. If you are myopic, take comfort in the fact that, on average, people with myopia are more intelligent than those without it.

Multiple Sclerosis

Multiple sclerosis (MS) is a rare, chronic, inflammatory disease of the central nervous system. It is an autoimmune disease; antibodies to myelin, the insulation around nerves, destroy the myelin in a patchy fashion. This leads to progressive, but variable, neurological dysfunction. Familial occurrence is uncommon. More females than males are affected.

There have been claims of association with a variety of infections, viral or bacterial, but the data are inconsistent. Claims that the frequency varies with latitude have been discredited.

MS is most prevalent in Caucasian persons of Northern European descent (two cases per thousand). In the United States, prevalence is about half this. Japan has a rate of only two cases per one hundred thousand, and MS is exceedingly rare in Africa. However, Americans of Japanese descent have a prevalence approximately one-quarter that of Caucasian Americans, and Americans of African descent have about one-third the prevalence of Caucasian Americans. These figures suggest both an environmental effect and genetic susceptibility.

The sib of a patient with MS has an increased chance, about 2%, of being affected, and about 5% if a parent is also affected, suggesting that genes have some role. Furthermore, an identical co-twin of an MS patient has about a 30% risk, as compared to about 5% for a non-identical twin.

The HLA gene and other genes associated with the immune system have small effects on susceptibility, but not enough to be useful for prognosis. There is also an association with the gene for basic myelin protein which, when clarified, may help improve understanding.

Neural Tube Defects (NTDs)

The brain and spinal cord develop from the embryonic neural tube, which arises when a flat plate of cells along the back of the very early embryo rolls up into a tube. If the tube fails to close at the head end, the brain is left open, and degenerates, resulting in anencephaly, in which much of the open brain has been destroyed. If the failure to close is lower down, there is an opening in the spinal cord (spina bifida); the cord may bulge onto the surface, and suffer damage.

Children with anencephaly die before or shortly after birth. Spina bifida may cause paralysis if the spinal cord is damaged, which may or may not be surgically correctible. Hydrocephalus (water on the brain) may be a complication. Most children with spina bifida who survive are handicapped to varying degrees.

NTDs result from the interaction of many genes and many environmental factors. There is progress in identifying some of the genes contributing to susceptibility. But the most dramatic progress has been the discovery that an environmental factor, folic acid, is important. For parents of children with either anencephaly or spina bifida, the next child has about one chance in twenty of having an NTD. But supplementing the mother's diet with folic acid in early pregnancy reduces this risk to less than 1%. It is recommended that all women of child-bearing age should take at least 0.4 milligrams of folic acid a day. Fortification of foods, such as flour, with folic acid has led to a substantial decrease in NTDs in various populations.

Prenatal diagnosis of NTDs can be done in several ways. An ultrasound examination will detect all cases of anencephaly and most cases of spina bifida. Secondly, there is a protein made by the fetal liver, alpha-fetoprotein (AFP), which normally leaks into the amniotic fluid in small amounts. If there is an abnormal opening in the fetus, such as a neural tube defect, much greater amounts of AFP leak into the amniotic fluid so that amniocentesis, and measurement of AFP in the amniotic fluid provides another means of diagnosis.

Furthermore, when there is a high AFP level in the amniotic fluid, there is also some increase in AFP in the mother's blood serum. Since this has resulted in a screening test that may be given routinely to pregnant women, I shall spend some time on it.

The distribution of AFP values in the mother's serum when there is a neural tube defect overlaps the normal distribution, so an elevated maternal serum AFP (MSAFP) is a warning that something may be wrong, not a diagnosis. Furthermore, there are several hormones, such as human chorionic gonadotropin and estriol, whose values are altered in maternal serum when the fetus has a chromosome problem. Many prenatal programs offer a "triple test," measuring a combination of AFP and two (or more) hormones in the mother's blood. Either a high value or a low value for any of the tests is an indication to consider further investigation. Abnormal values are found in about 5% of pregnancies. It should be emphasized that an abnormal finding for any of these compounds is only an indication that there is a chance that something is wrong, and that further investigation is indicated. Consult your nearest genetic counselor if you are concerned.

Obesity

Our bodies are made up mainly of water, protein, and fat. A certain amount of fat is necessary, but as the proportion of fat increases we become overweight. When it extends well beyond the normal range we call it obesity. Besides being a nuisance (altered clothes, negative self-image), being overweight is a health hazard. The fatter one is, the higher the risk for a variety of diseases, including heart disease, high-blood pressure (and thus stroke), diabetes, gallstones, and cancer. Obesity is said to be second only to smoking as a preventable cause of death in the United States. Furthermore, obese women have an increased risk for neural tube defects in their children.

Obesity is a disorder of fat cells (adipocytes), the cells distributed throughout the body that store fat. It can result from either an increase in the number of fat cells or an increase in the amount of fat in the fat cells. It is thought that the number and size of the baby's fat cells are programmed during late pregnancy and early infancy, so it is important to keep infants from becoming overweight.

The regulation of body weight is very complex. It involves many players, including the hypothalamus in the brain, the hormone-producing glands (pituitary, thyroid, adrenal, and pancreas), the intestines, and the fat cells.

The hypothalamus is the control center. It sends signals to the various other organs to turn on or shut off hormone production. It probably also acts as a "hunger" center and a "satiety" center. On cue, hormones are released from organs, to target receptors in other organs. These organs produce other hormones that act as feedback responses to the original organs or stimulate still other organs or cells. The sympathetic nervous system responds to dietary excess by increasing energy expenditure. This intricate system of checks and balances responds to the intake of calories in the food and the output of calories by exercise. All of the hormones and receptors are proteins, each one the product of a gene, so there is lots of opportunity for genes to be involved with weight control. Some of the genes have been identified. I will not attempt to describe the system in detail, but will give one illustrative example: the leptin gene.

Leptin was discovered in the mouse—one of several mouse obesity genes that have been identified at the DNA level. The Human Genome Project revealed the same DNA sequence in people. The gene product, leptin, is produced by the fat cells. Loss of fat decreases leptin output, which tells the brain that the body needs calories and to please send hunger signals to the appropriate organs. Increased food intake increases fat, and increases leptin output, which tells the brain to reduce food intake. It's more complicated than that, and leptin acts in many other ways as well, but that is the general idea.

When the leptin gene was first discovered, it was thought that mutations in it or the leptin receptor gene might be important in causing human obesity. In fact, they account for a very small proportion of obese patients. But knowing the structure of the leptin molecule may lead to the design of drugs that will counteract obesity.

Obviously, there are many genes that can predispose to obesity; in the geneticist's jargon, obesity is genetically heterogeneous. For purposes of discussion, the various types of obesity can be put into three classes: obesity syndromes, resistant obesity, and multifactorial obesity.

Obesity syndromes are conditions where the obesity is associated with other abnormalities such as mental retardation, and malformations. Many of them are caused by mutant genes; they are all rare, so I will say no more about them.

Resistant obesity is the type that is so hard to treat. Patients go on rigorous exercise programs and starvation diets. They may consent to having tucks taken in their stomachs, or even having their jaws sewn together to reduce food intake. They may manage to lose some weight, but often relapse after some months. There is a strong genetic basis, and a few specific genes have been identified. Understanding what these genes are doing will lead to the design of better drugs. These may be directed at reducing appetite, reducing fat storage by speeding up metabolism, or preventing the formation of fat cells. As the Human Genome Project progresses, more genes will surely be found, and new drugs will be designed without the dangerous side effects shown by some already released and withdrawn from the market.

Multifactorial obesity is the most prevalent type, resulting simply from eating too much and exercising too little—aided, no doubt, by a genetic constitution that predisposes to weight gain. A small change in the balance between calorie intake in the food and output with exercise can lead to an insidious progression towards fattiness. Choosing high-calorie fast foods to save time, and using the time saved to watch television instead of going for a run or a walk, can be the first step on the path to fattiness. The best way to avoid or correct this cultural obesity is by eating less and exercising more. But if this fails, partially or completely, there may be a need for drugs.

This kind of obesity certainly runs in families, and studies of twins and adopted children show that genes play a major role. Mapping of genes predisposing to obesity is proceeding rapidly. Over a dozen such genes have been mapped, and several have been identified. Their study will, no doubt, improve understanding of how the system works, and point the way to better treatments.

If you have a fat relative, how likely are you to be fat? Most family studies do not separate resistant from multifactorial obesity, so it is hard to find good data. Perhaps it is sufficient to say that your risk is definitely increased, and more so the more fat relatives you have, and the fatter they are, particularly if they were fat as children.

There is a serious epidemic of obesity that needs urgent attention. It involves most of the world. A recent survey found that 61% of Americans are overweight, if not actually obese—a sharp increase in the past two decades. The results of obesity are already making heavy demands on our health-care system, in terms of more heart disease, stroke, cancer, and the rest. This epidemic is not of the resistant kind of obesity. It is clearly not due to changes in gene frequencies, but in lifestyle—fast foods, TV instead of exercise, and so on. A program of public education and pressure is required to reverse it. If nothing is done, we will pay a heavy price in health care costs and reduced life span.

Parkinson Disease (PD)

Parkinson disease (PD) is a progressive neurological disorder. Patients have resting tremor, muscular rigidity, slow movements, postural instability, and perhaps dementia. The disease results from degeneration of neurons in a part of the brain (the substantia nigra) that produces an important neurotransmitter, dopamine. The average age of onset is about sixty, and it affects about 1% of those over that age.

A number of environmental factors have been invoked, with varying degrees of certainty, as contributing to PD. Increased risks have been reported for farmers, rural dwellers, drinkers of well water, those with head trauma, and those exposed to pesticides, herbicides, and industrial pollutants. But there are conflicting findings, and no particular agent has been identified except for certain drugs. A variety of neurotoxic chemicals can play a role, but what decides who, among exposed people, gets it? There is evidence that genetic differences in the enzymes that break down these environmental toxins may alter susceptibility. Impaired breakdown would mean increased exposure.

The search for susceptibility genes is progressing. In a few families, major genes are the culprit. Six or more major Parkinson genes have been identified, all rare. Understanding how they act may help in understanding the disease, and designing better drugs. For the rest, PD certainly seems to be familial, but there is no clear family pattern. At least six loci that cause a modest increase in susceptibility have been mapped, including some that influence age of onset. Excluding the major gene families, the frequency of PD in sibs of patients is around 5%.

The bottom line is that PD is a multifactorial disorder. If you have a parent or sib with PD, your risk of getting it before you die of old age may be increased somewhat. If you have more than one affected relative, your risk may be higher. Irrespective of your family history, it is wise not to expose yourself unduly to insecticides, herbicides, or other industrial chemicals.

Psoriasis

Psoriasis is a chronic skin disease that affects about 2% of the population. It is characterized by itchy, red, scaly skin patches, usually found on the scalp, elbows, and knees, and may be associated with severe arthritis. The usual age of onset is between fifteen and thirty years old.

The condition is very familial, and the inheritance is probably multifactorial, involving at least several genes, plus environmental factors such as streptococcal infections and stress.

Several susceptibility genes have been mapped, one of them close to the HLA gene cluster, which is involved with immunity.

If one parent has psoriasis, the lifetime risk for each child is about 25%. If both parents are affected, the risk goes up to 65%. For the sib of a psoriatic person with unaffected parents, the risk is at least 10%.

Restless Legs Syndrome

This is a fairly common condition, affecting 5% or more of the population, who have uncomfortable and unpleasant sensations in the legs that appear at rest, inducing an irresistible desire to move them. The symptoms are worse in the evening or at night than during the day, and are partially or totally relieved by movement. Most patients experience sleep disturbances. There seems to be some connection with Parkinsonism. Patients with Parkinson disease have an increased frequency of restless leg syndrome. Furthermore, the condition can be treated with certain drugs that are used for Parkinson disease.

In some families, particularly those with an onset before age thirty, the cause of the syndrome is a major dominant gene—one that has its effect when present in a single dose. Several genes increasing susceptibility have been mapped. Identifying them, and what they do, may improve our understanding of Parkinson disease.

Scoliosis, Adolescent

In children with idiopathic (cause unknown) scoliosis, the spine has a structurally-fixed lateral curvature with a rotatory component. It occurs in about four per thousand girls, and much less often in boys. Twin studies suggest a genetic component, but little is known of its nature. The risk for first-degree relatives is about 5%.

Sex Chromosome Abnormalities (SCAs)

Females have two X chromosomes; males have an X and a Y. Extra or missing sex chromosomes cause far less trouble than abnormalities of the other chromosomes. The Y chromosome has very few genes on it other than those that decide that the embryo will be male. The four most common sex chromosome abnormalities are: males with an extra X, or 47, XXY Klinefelter syndrome; females with an extra X, or 47, XXX syndrome; females with a missing X, or 45, XO Turner syndrome; and males with an extra Y, or 47, XYY syndrome.

Sex chromosome abnormalities affect about one in four hundred newborn children, and in mid-pregnancy the frequency may be as high as one in two hundred fifty; many of them die before birth. In the early days the children with SCAs who were described in the literature were often severely affected children in institutions, since they were the ones who got to have their chromosomes examined. This gave a very bad impression of what it meant to be a child with an SCA. Proposals to screen newborns for SCAs, and follow them throughout childhood to get an unbiased picture of their development were vigorously opposed by those who thought it would be unethical. They feared that it would stigmatize the children, and that the very fact of being followed would alter their development. The result was that parents of children with SCAs could not be provided with accurate information about the outlook for their child's development, and often got unduly pessimistic forecasts. It is only now that an unbiased picture is emerging, at least for the four most common ones, from multi-center, long-term studies of individuals followed from birth.

The four groups differ from one another in various ways, but have certain features in common. The bottom line is that the outlook is much better than had been thought. They are all at some risk for mild speech/language and motor delays and learning disabilities. They have IQs mostly in the normal range, with a mean ten to fifteen points lower than that of their sibs. They all have normal adult adaptation. See the entries for the particular conditions for more details about their specific characteristics.

Since these chromosomal problems result from mistakes in separation of the chromosomes when the egg or sperm are forming, the risk that a subsequent child of the same parents will be affected is very small.

45 XO (Turner) syndrome

Of the four common sex chromosome syndromes, girls with Turner syndrome, in which one X-chromosome is missing, show the most severe developmental problems—some so severe that they cause death before birth. The frequency at birth is about one in two thousand females.

Surviving girls with Turner syndrome are short, may have webbing of the skin at the neck, and other minor anomalies. There may be malformations of the heart or kidneys. Their ovaries degenerate before puberty, so they are sterile. Treatment with growth hormone, and estrogen at puberty may be helpful, though not for their sterility.

Their intelligence is usually in the normal range, but average about ten to fifteen IQ points lower than that of their sibs. They are at risk for mild speech and learning disabilities and may have spatial relations problems. Many of them go through life undiagnosed.

47 XXX syndrome

About one in every thousand girls is born with an extra X-chromosome. They tend to be tall and thin, and have good general health, so they, too, are often not diagnosed. They are at risk for mild speech and learning disabilities. Their IQs are in the normal range, but average ten to fifteen points lower than those of their sibs.

47 XXY Klinefelter syndrome

Klinefelter syndrome, 47 XXY, is the most common genetic cause of human male infertility, with a frequency of about one in six hundred males. It occurs in about 12% of azoospermic (having no sperm) men. As with Down syndrome, Klinefelter syndrome occurs more often in the children of older mothers.

The syndrome is very variable. Klinefelter males are tall and may have a feminine body build; some will have enlargement of the breasts (gynecomastia). The testes are small and produce few sperm or, more often, none at all. Testosterone therapy at puberty may help, but will not prevent the gynecomastia or restore fertility.

XXY children may have mild speech/language and motor delays, and learning disabilities. They have IQs in the normal range, but average about ten to fifteen points lower than their sibs. They have pleasant personalities.

Advances in reproductive technology have allowed some males with Klinefelter syndrome to have children with the aid of intracytoplasmic sperm injection (ICSI) and *in vitro* fertilization. In ICSI sperm is injected directly into an egg, which is then put into the uterus. Klinefelter men have, as expected, an increased frequency (about 5%) of XX and XY sperm, but also an increase in disomy 21 (an extra chromosome 21), so there is, theoretically, an increased risk of Down syndrome in a child of a Klinefelter man conceived by ICSI. There are not enough data to see if this is actually so.

47 XYY syndrome

About one in one thousand boys has an extra Y chromosome. These children tend to be tall, and to have good physical health. They are fertile. They may have mild speech/language and motor delays, and some have learning problems. They may be prone to childhood temper tantrums, but not to aggression. They do not have a predisposition to criminality, as the popular press used to claim, sometimes referring to the Y as a "criminal chromosome." See Criminality in the next chapter for the story. Their school performance in general is good. Their IQ distribution is about ten points lower than that of their sibs, but in the normal range.

Spina Bifida—see Neural Tube Defects

Squint—see Strabismus

Strabismus

Strabismus is a condition where the two eyes do not look in the same direction. There can be divergent (exophoria) and convergent (esophoria) strabismus. It occurs in 3 to 5% of children, depending on the population and diagnostic criteria.

Studies of the genetics of strabismus have not come up with any clear-cut results because of differing diagnostic criteria and genetic heterogeneity. No single mechanism, environmental agent, or gene defect has been identified. Identical (monozygotic) twins are more likely to be concordant (both affected) than fraternal (dizygotic) pairs, and near relatives are much more likely to be affected than non-relatives, so there are genetic factors involved, but there are no precise risk figures to use for genetic counseling. Here are some imprecise figures: for unaffected parents with an affected child, the chance that the next child will be affected is about 15%; for an affected parent with an affected child, the chance for the next child is about 40%.

Maternal smoking and low birth weight are (perhaps related) environmental risk factors, but not very strong ones.

Stuttering

In the speech of those who stutter there are involuntary repetitions, lengthened sounds, or arrests of sounds. Stuttering occurs in about 5% of children aged three to five years. It goes away by puberty in most children, but persists in about 1%.

The biological basis of stuttering is unknown. Recent research suggests that stutterers have poor connections between various areas of the brain relevant to speech.

Childhood stuttering affects about twice as many boys as girls; in adults it is about five times as many. Family and twin studies suggest a genetic predisposition, with many genes involved, possibly including a major locus increasing liability. If you stutter, your children are more likely to stutter, but how much more likely is not known. Maybe some specific genes will be identified some day, and the situation will become clearer.

Turner Syndrome—see Sex Chromosome Abnormalities

Varicose Veins

Varicose veins are probably the most common vascular abnormality. They are usually caused by venous congestion due to long standing. The chronic increase in pressure causes the vein to dilate so the valves (that prevent back flow) become incompetent. The venous blood backs up leading to swollen veins and poor circulation. Mine developed when I was in third-year medicine and spent a lot of time standing around bedsides and operating tables. An old Danish study showed that they do run in the family in a multifactorial pattern. A recent British twin study showed that they have a prevalence of close to 25%, and the concordance rates suggest that both genetic and environmental factors are important. There is linkage to at least one chromosome region on chromosome 16.

4

Genetics of Behavior: Normal and Abnormal

Behavior is an exceedingly complex affair, and it follows that its genetics will be complex. Progress in genetic analysis is slow, and for almost all the behavioral traits I will talk about, I'll say much the same thing. Twin studies and adoption studies show that genes are involved to some extent. Environmental influences are also important. Geneticists are searching for the relevant genes but are not having much success. In fact, they are probably doing better at finding behavioral genes in dogs and mice than in people.

This chapter will discuss, in alphabetical order, selected behavioral traits, including: normal behavioral traits and personality; abnormal behavior, such as alcoholism, criminality, and the obsessive-compulsive disorders, and the psychoses—the depressive disorders and schizophrenia.

Alcoholism

Alcoholism is an addiction to ethyl alcohol with its well-known consequences. That alcoholism runs in families has been recognized since the days of Plato, but how and why are far from clear. Animal studies have shown that genes influence alcohol tolerance and preference, but no alcoholism genes have been identified.

Twin studies and adoption studies of alcoholism suggest a moderate genetic influence, particularly in men. One Swedish study divides alcoholics into two types. Type 2 occurs predominantly in men; they have an early-onset, moderate alcohol dependence, and are likely to have social and legal problems. In type 1, dependence can be mild or severe. It occurs in both men and women, and has a later onset, fewer social and legal problems, and less evidence of a genetic influence than type 2. This concept has been criticized by some as oversimplified and implausible, so there is need for clarification.

As with other behavioral traits, there have been searches for relevant genes. There will be found, no doubt, several such genes, of small effect, increasing the probability that their carriers will become alcoholic, particularly in an unfavorable environment.

One of the most clear-cut examples of a gene influencing alcoholism is one that reduces the predisposition. After alcohol is consumed, it is converted by the enzyme alcohol dehydrogenase (ADH) to acetaldehyde, which is further broken down by the enzyme aldehyde dehydrogenase (ALDH). If the ALDH is deficient, the acetaldehyde piles up in the blood, and produces facial flushing and other unpleasant effects of intoxication. Those who carry a mutant, inactive form of the ALDH gene are deterred from drinking alcohol by these unpleasant effects, and are unlikely to become alcoholic. The mutant ALDH is much more frequent in Asians than Caucasians, which may account, at least in part, for their lower frequency of alcoholism.

For an individual family it may be best simply to recognize that there are various risk factors (in addition to not being Asian), one of the strongest being to have a parent or sib with alcoholism that started at an early age, and was associated with adolescent antisocial behavior. In that case, it would be wise to watch for signs of the predisposition in family members, and try to provide a protective environment.

Attention Deficit-Hyperactivity Disorder (ADHD)

Attention deficit-hyperactivity disorder (ADHD) is the most common childhood behavioral disorder; it affects about 5 or 10% of children and adolescents, and about 3% of adults. Persistent inattention and/or hyperactive-impulsive behavior lead to impaired social and/or academic functioning. Boys are affected about four times as often as girls.

The condition is certainly familial—sibs of an ADHD patient have a five-fold increase in risk. Heritability is estimated as 60 to 80%. There is some connection with other psychiatric disorders and with autism and dyslexia. The situation is very confused. The search is on for relevant genes. When these have been identified, the picture will, no doubt, become much clearer.

Criminality

The causes of criminality, and the antisocial behavior that leads to it, are exceedingly complex. Obviously, there is a large environmental component. If there is a genetic component to the tendency to transgress the law—and get caught—it is, no doubt, related to personality traits such as aggressiveness and intelligence, which are genetically influenced. So it is not surprising that twin studies and adoption studies of criminality show some evidence of a genetic influence and a large environmental component.

Adoption studies show that the two interact. When children of parents with a low-crime record were adopted by parents with a high-crime record, they showed only a small increase in criminality—presumably their genes were protective in a criminal environment. When children of parents with a high-crime record were adopted by low-crime parents, they also had low criminality scores—presumably because their environment was protective. But children of parents with a high-crime record adopted by high-crime parents had a high criminality score. This suggests that when children who inherit genes predisposing to criminality are raised in a low-crime environment, the criminality genes are not expressed. But in a high-crime environment, the criminal predisposition is fulfilled. The message is, improve the environment and disable the crime genes.

A recent Australian study will, if confirmed, provide a beautiful example of such a gene-environment interaction. It involves an enzyme, monoamine oxidase A (MAOA), which inactivates neurotransmitters such as serotonin and dopamine. Low levels of the enzyme have been linked to aggression. The MAOA gene, on the X-chromosome, exists in two forms, one with low- and the other with high-MAOA activity. The study showed that abuse in childhood increased the frequency of antisocial behavior in young adulthood, mostly in males with the low form of the MAOA gene. The 12% of males with low activity accounted for 44% of the violent convictions. Perhaps this will pave the way to preventive drug treatment for abused children with low MAOA, but not, I hope, at the expense of measures to reduce child abuse.

That is all I will say about the genetics of criminality, except for one example that has attracted a lot of public attention, namely the so-called criminal chromosome which turned out not to be criminal at all.

Here is the story of the "criminal chromosome," as best I can recollect it:

In the early days after human chromosomes became countable, there was a Scottish geneticist, Patricia Jacobs, who wondered if having a Y-chromosome (the male-determining one) was the reason that males are, on average, taller than females. If this were so, XYY men should be taller than XY men. To test this hypothesis one should look at Y-chromosome number in a group of tall men. Where to find a large group of tall men? How about a prison, where a sample of tall volunteers might be easily available? This was arranged, and the group of tall men did, indeed, contain more XYY men than expected. Since these men were in trouble with the law, this did not necessarily mean that XYY men were criminally disposed. But some members of the press jumped to this fallacious conclusion, and there was much talk of the criminal chromosome. Lawyers pled that XYY clients were not to blame for their actions since it was in their genes. Obviously, more information was needed. Plans to screen newborns for XYY and follow them to assess the effects of the extra Y were blocked, on the grounds that knowing that a boy was XYY would be prejudicial to him. This, of course, made it much more difficult to get an answer.

When the dust settled, it seemed clear that XYY males did indeed occur more frequently in prisoners than in the general population, for reasons that are still not clear. But this was a minority of all XYY males, and those in prison were there largely for non-violent crimes. On average, they have slightly lower than average IQ's. But the main message is that there a lot of XYY men who do very well in life, most of whom will never know they have an extra Y chromosome.

I know one mother of a baby boy who had unexpectedly been found to be XYY when prenatal diagnosis was done to screen for Down syndrome. She came to plead—nay demand—that the record be destroyed. She was afraid that, when her son was running for prime minister, some nosy reporter would discover his record and brand him as criminally disposed. He was a beautiful little boy. I wonder how he made out.

Personality

How often do we hear someone say "you are just like your mother" or father. Usually this refers to personality or temperament, and all too often it is not meant as a compliment. Are human personality traits inherited? Well, different breeds of dogs have different personalities, and these are largely inherited, so why not people? Some aspects of personality appear very early in life (some psychologists say even before birth, before the environment has a chance to act), suggesting that they may have a genetic basis. And children are more like their parents than non-relatives in their patterns of social behavior, i.e. their personality. But, as in the case of physical traits, they may differ sharply. How much of the resemblance is due to "nature" (genes), and how much to "nurture" (environment) has been debated since the days of Francis Galton, in the late 19th century, with the eugenicists (pro nature) on one side and most psychologists and psychiatrists (pro nurture) on the other. As knowledge of our genome increases, the muddy waters are beginning to clear, but only a little. Why have the waters been so muddy?

For one thing, behavioral traits are much harder to define, and measure, than physical ones. It is much easier to measure the length of a person's arm or their blood pressure, than their sensitivity or their aggressiveness. Psychologists have been getting better at breaking down personality into more specific traits such as introversion/extroversion, impulsiveness, extravagance, anxiousness, passiveness, aggressiveness, and so on, and measuring them. This should lead to progress in defining the genetic contribution.

A second difficulty is that genetic studies are harder when traits cannot be sharply classified as present or absent. Genetic studies of normal behavior are difficult, because most behavioral characteristics are classified as more or less, not present or absent; they are continuous. Therefore, if there is a genetic basis for a behavioral trait, it must be complex. That is why much of behavior genetics is statistical, involving correlations, twin studies, and heritability estimates, rather than pedigree studies and Mendelian ratios.

As I said, psychologists have been busy classifying behavior into specific components, such as introversion/extroversion, neuroticism, aggression, novelty seeking, and many others. They have been developing tests for these traits, so that individuals can be measured, and compared with their relatives and non-relatives for specific personality traits. How much the trait in question is influenced by genes is measured by how much people resemble their relatives, how much more similar identical twins are than fraternal twins, and how much more adopted children resemble their biological than their adoptive parents.

Twin studies have discovered some remarkable cases of identical twins reared apart who were astonishingly similar. A pair raised apart, and unknown to each other, might find that they both were firemen, had Western moustaches, smoked the same brand of cigarettes, drank the same brand of beer, had wives with the same name, two children, with the same names, and so on. This would suggest an important role for genes, but remember that these were only a few of thousands of pairs. Could this be coincidence? Some identical pairs, even when reared together, turn out to be rather different. I know of one pair of brothers who are very similar in appearance and mannerisms. One was a famous geneticist and the other a distinguished juror, even though they were raised together. One needs to look at similarities and differences in a large sample of twin pairs, not just the unusual ones.

Twin studies have shown that almost all of the personality traits studied showed heritabilities of 30 to 50%—i.e., genes account for less than half of the variation in the trait, but certainly have some influence.

Granted that genes influence our behavior, *which* genes, and how do they act? The neuro-biochemists tell us that the way our brains function, including our temperaments and moods, depends on a group of chemicals called neurotransmitters. The rates at which these chemicals are produced in certain areas of the brain, transported to other areas, taken up by receptors, and recycled, or broken down, influence their effects on the brain. These processes depend on enzymes and other proteins that, of course, are controlled by genes, so it would be very surprising if genes did not affect brain function. But they do so in very complex ways. Neuro-geneticists have begun the process of sorting out which genes are involved, how they function, and under what circumstances, but progress is slow, findings are often conflicting, and conclusions tentative. A number of personality traits have been tentatively linked to particular places on a chromosome (mapped). No doubt some of the associations being found will turn out to be real, but no one gene accounts for more than about 5% of the variation. That is, they are minor differences, so they will not be of much use to identify people that are susceptible to personality disorders, before they get sick. So don't worry about there ever being prenatal diagnosis to eliminate neurotic people!

Psychoses

The major psychoses are so common that almost all of us have had personal experience of them either in ourselves, our families, or our friends and acquaintances. There are two major groups: the affective disorders,—manic-depressive psychosis (bipolar), and cyclic depression (unipolar),—and schizophrenia.

Affective disorders
Manic-depressive (bipolar) disorder. At least 2% of us will develop a bipolar, or manic-depressive, disorder at some point in our lives. Manic-depressives alternate

between periods of depression and periods of mania—intense activity and euphoria. The depressions may be severe—up to 10 or 20 % of those affected take their own lives. The manic episodes may be periods of intense creativity. Think of Vincent van Gogh, William Blake, Walt Whitman, T. S. Eliot, and lots of others.

Family, twin, and adoptive studies all suggest that genes are important in determining susceptibility to bipolar depressive disorders, but that environmental factors are also involved. Much effort has been put into mapping susceptibility genes, with conflicting and confusing results. Several genes have been mapped, including one associated with HLA (of the immune system) and one on the X-chromosome. There may be a subtype in which the mania is mild. There may also be genetic differences in the way patients handle anti-depressant drugs.

Patients with *schizoaffective disorder* have symptoms of both depressive disorder and schizophrenia, suggesting a genetic connection between the two, the nature of which remains unclear. A gene has been found that is linked to both disorders, which may help to explain the connection.

Unipolar disorders, or cyclical depressions without manic episodes, are probably less severe forms of the bipolar disorder. Combined results of a number of studies suggest that sibs or children of a person with bipolar depression have about a 9% chance of having a bipolar depression themselves, and a 14% chance of having a unipolar depression. For persons with a unipolar depression, the risk for a sib or child is about 2% for bipolar, and 14% for unipolar depression.

No environmental factors have been identified as yet, but the disease seems to be affecting more people, and at an earlier age. Could this be a sign of our increasingly stressful life-styles?

As for specific genes, there are some tentative associations with genes involved in neurotransmission. A predisposition gene on chromosome 12 is expressed particularly in males. Evidence is beginning to accumulate for genes that predispose to depression in people who are exposed to environmental insults.

If, thanks to the Human Genome Project, some predisposing genes are actually found, and their modes of action identified, that may open the way to designing better anti-depressant drugs, and identifying which patients respond best to which drugs. I hope so.

Schizophrenia

The prototype of schizophrenia is a young adult who starts having delusions, hallucinations, disordered thinking and concentration, erratic behavior, and severely inappropriate emotional responses. Each of us has, on average, about one chance in one hundred of having it. If we have a schizophrenic parent or sib, does that increase the chance? Yes it does. Does that mean it's genetic? Not necessarily, but there is now evidence that genes have a lot to do with it.

If you have a schizophrenic brother, sister, or parent, you have about a 10% chance of getting it, a tenfold increase. (But of course this chance decreases the longer you live without it.) If you have both a schizophrenic sib and parent, your chance is about 16%. But couldn't this be because you live in a schizophrenic environment? Possibly, but both twin and adoption studies argue against this. Monozygotic (identical) twins are much more often both affected (around 45%) than are dizygotic (fraternal) pairs (15%), even when they are separated at birth and raised in different families. The figures suggest that genes account for between 63 and 85% of the variation.

Children of schizophrenic parents adopted by non-schizophrenic parents are no less likely to become schizophrenic than if they had not been adopted, so the environment does not seem to help reduce their risk much.

There has been a lot of progress in sorting out the neurochemical basis of this disorder. Several neurotransmitters have been implicated, including dopamine, serotonin, and glutamate, and drug development is aimed at them or their receptors. These are, of course, under genetic control, and their genes are likely candidates for susceptibility genes. So far, attempts to find specific genes predisposing to schizophrenia have been discouraging. There appear to be several genes—perhaps as many as twelve or more. Some of them will no doubt be identified, thanks to the Human Genome Project, but each will increase susceptibility by only a small amount. Don't expect any gene therapy.

As for environmental factors, it was thought that living with a schizophrenic might drive a person towards schizophrenia (folie a deux), as might having a distant or manipulative parent, but the twin and adoption studies do not support this. The disease seems to have roots in the development of the nervous system, and some of the environmental factors may act through these roots. There are anatomical differences in the brains of schizophrenics, suggesting defects in migration of neurons during development. Schizophrenics are more likely to be born in the winter months, suggesting that prenatal events, such as maternal infections may be involved. Folic acid deficiency, both before and after birth may predispose to schizophrenia. Brain damage during birth is another possible factor. All in all, environmental predisposing factors seem to be just as elusive as the genetic ones.

Obsessive-Compulsive Disorder

Obsessive-compulsive disorder is a chronic, disabling disorder with a frequency of around 3%. Patients have intrusive thoughts or images (obsessions), which increase anxiety, and they make repetitive or ritualistic actions (compulsions) to decrease anxiety.

Family and twin studies indicate that genetic factors influence susceptibility, and there is some overlap with Tourette syndrome (childhood onset of motor and vocal tics and behavioral abnormalities). There is so much confusion that, until things have been sorted out, all I can say is that, if you have a first-degree relative with OCD, you have an increased risk (around 10%) of having it too, especially if the relative had a childhood onset.

Suicidal Behavior

Of course there are no "suicide genes" as such, but there do seem to be genes that increase the chance that their carriers will commit suicide. There is enough evidence for this that a recent issue of the American Journal of Medical Genetics (vol. 133C (1)) is devoted to the subject. As one might expect, the situation is complicated.

In developed countries, the lifetime prevalence of suicide runs around 3 or 4 % (though there are differences between countries), and the incidence is increasing. Family, twin, and adoption studies all demonstrate that there are genetic predisposing factors (55% of the variation) and environmental factors (45%)—that is, genes and environment are about equally involved. Even when predisposing factors such as mood disorders, schizophrenia, and drug abuse are taken into account, there still seems to be a specific genetic predisposition. Work is just beginning on the tremendous task of sorting out the genes that predispose to those personality traits that increase the risk of suicide, such as impulsivity, neuroticism and anxiety-related traits; aggression and anger-related traits; hopelessness; low self-esteem; and childhood trauma. It will be a long time before any specific genes are identified.

In practical terms, for any first-degree relative of people who killed themselves, or attempted to do so, the risk of suicidal attempts is increased about four-fold, to 12 to 16 % over their lifetime. So having a suicidal near-relative should be considered a warning.

Conclusion

I hope you have now gained some appreciation of how important genes are for your habitus, health, and happiness, and how paying attention to your family tree may tell you something, though of course not everything, about your own genes and health prospects. Sir William Osler advised us to choose our parents wisely, but not only are you unable to choose your parents, but you cannot choose which of their genes you draw. You get only half of your mother's genes and half of your father's. This is why you resemble your parents and sibs in some respects but not others.

You have also seen that genes do not determine our characteristics by themselves—environmental factors are important too. Although you have no control over the assortment of parental genes that fate dealt you, you do have at least some control over your lifestyle and that of your children. This book has aimed at helping you see how to adjust your lifestyle to guard against the particular risks that your family tree says you are subject to.

A recurrent theme of the book is that the common familial disorders are caused by a combination of several genes, each with a small effect, and several environmental factors. Each one increases your susceptibility to the disorder, and if you draw enough of them, you get sick. Because each factor has a relatively small effect, they are hard to sort out, identify, and measure.

The new techniques of DNA technology are identifying more and more mutant genes that contribute to disease. Most of them are those with a major effect, because they are easier to find. They cause diseases showing Mendelian inheritance, and most are so rare that you have probably never heard of them; they are beyond the scope of this book. It is more difficult to identify the mutant genes of small effect that contribute to susceptibility for the common familial disorders. But more and more of these are also being identified. Furthermore, techniques for detecting the mutant genes will become less expensive. There are now microarrays that make it possible to test a thousand or more of a person's genes on a chip no bigger than your thumb nail!

Researchers are pursuing not only the susceptibility genes for the common disorders, but also the environmental factors with which they interact. There are several ongoing studies in which tens of thousands of families are typed for thousands of genes, and also for hundreds of factors in their environments. These families are then followed for many years to see what diseases they develop. In this way, the connections between diseases, genes, and environments will be unraveled, but it will take many years.

Some enthusiasts foresee a world in which everyone will be screened at birth for thousands of genes, that will tell us not only which diseases we will surely develop (hemophilia, sickle-cell anemia, Huntington disease), but also what diseases we will be susceptible to if we choose the wrong lifestyle, and which drugs we should take when we do get a disease. As the Bard might have written, O brave new world that hath such wonders in it!

But geneticists are beginning to think that this view is a bit unrealistic. We already offer testing for many genes, such as the Huntington disease gene, and the BRCA gene for breast cancer, but only to people at high risk, who have received genetic counseling before and after testing. Whether to be tested is not a simple decision. Some people choose not to be tested; they prefer not to know. For both ethical and economic reasons, genetic testing is not likely ever to be done on a population-wide basis.

Testing for mutant genes will be useful for predicting how we will react to drugs, and for increasing our understanding of disease. But, for a long time, the best indicator of what diseases we are susceptible to, and what lifestyles will guard against them, will be our family histories. Know your family tree

Glossary

Adoption studies: studies that measure whether adopted children are more like their biological parents than their adoptive parents with respect to a given trait. If they are, that is strong evidence that the trait is genetically influenced.

Alleles: alternative forms of a gene.

Alpha-feto protein (AFP): a protein produced by the fetal liver, which normally stays within the fetus. If there is an abnormal opening in the fetus, such as a neural tube defect, large amounts of AFP get into the amniotic fluid, which can be used for diagnosis. Some AFP also gets into the maternal serum, which can be used as a screening test.

Amino acids: the building blocks of protein. The sequence of amino acids in a protein determines its structure, and thereby its function.

Antibody: a protein that recognizes and combines with an antigen, sometimes with undesirable (allergic) side effects.

Antigen: any substance (usually a protein) that the body's immune system recognizes by producing an antibody that combines with it.

Base pairs: the four nitrogenous bases of DNA: guanine (G), cytosine (C), adenine (A), and thymine (T). G pairs only with C, and A with T. See also DNA.

Chromosomes: the carriers of the genes. Microscopically visible, thread-like bodies consisting of long strands of DNA in a protein framework. Humans have twenty-three pairs, one of each pair from each parent.

DNA: deoxyribonucleic acid, the genetic material. A rope-ladder-like structure in which the ropes are sugar-phosphate chains, and the steps are pairs of nucleotide bases (GC and AT). The sequence of base pairs at a particular place in the DNA contains the genetic information for the synthesis of the corresponding protein. That is, that particular DNA sequence is the gene for the protein.

Down syndrome: named after Langdon Down, an English physician, who first described it. This syndrome results from the presence of an extra chromosome 21 (trisomy 21). There is a characteristic facial appearance, mental retardation, and an increased frequency of heart and other malformations. These are happy children who love music. The IQ, on average, is about fifty points below that predicted from their parents' IQs.

Enzyme: a protein that catalyzes a specific biochemical reaction.

Familial: refers to a trait that occurs more often in the near relatives of a person with the trait than in those of persons without it.

Family studies: studies to measure whether a given trait occurs more often in the relatives of people who have the trait than in the general population. If the trait is not familial it is probably not genetic. If it is familial, further studies (see twin studies, adoption studies) are done to see whether this is for genetic or environmental reasons, or what combination of the two.

Gametes: eggs and sperm, the precursors of the next generation.

Gene: the basic unit of inheritance. The existence of genes was inferred by Mendel from the results of crosses in the garden pea. It is now known that the gene for a particular protein is a stretch of DNA that contains the information coded in its base pair sequence, that determines the amino acid sequence of that protein, and therefore its structure and function.

Genetic marker: a genetic difference, such as a blood group or a difference in a DNA base pair (SNP). If the marker's chromosomal location is known, the marker can be used to map the position of disease genes—see linkage.

Genetic screening: testing of groups of people to detect those at increased risk for having, or having a child with, a genetic disorder.

Genome: the entire genetic information of an organism. The human genome is the DNA of the set of twenty-three chromosomes and the mitochondrial DNA.

Haplotype: a pattern of DNA markers in a particular region of DNA that serves as its signature and can be traced through families or ethnic groups.

Heritability: a measure of the genetic contribution to the variability in a trait. See also twin studies.

Human Genome Project: a massive international project that succeeded in establishing the sequence of all three billion base pairs of the human DNA, and thus the genetic information contained in all twenty-three human chromosomes. It took thirteen years and cost well over a billion dollars.

Knock out mouse: a mouse which, by genetic engineering, has had a particular gene inactivated. They have become valuable models for the study of genetic disease.

Linkage: a measure of how close two genes are to each other on the chromosome. When the sperm and egg are forming, the maternal and paternal members of a pair of chromosomes exchange material, the process of recombination. This tends to separate genes on the same chromosome as they pass from one generation to the next. The closer together genes are the more they will not be separated, but stay together from one generation to the next—they are more closely linked.

Locus: the place on a chromosome where a gene is located.

Mendel: the Austrian monk who, from his studies of how traits segregated in the garden pea, demonstrated the ratios known as the Mendelian laws. These led him to propose that there were "heredity factors," later named genes, that maintained their identities from one generation to the next.

Mendelian trait: a trait that runs in families according to the Mendelian laws, which predict characteristic patterns of inheritance. If a trait follows these laws, it is controlled by a difference in a single gene.

Mitochondria: sacs in the cytoplasm of a cell, which contain enzymes for the conversion of nutrients to energy—the power house of the cell. They contain a special, circular DNA. They do not occur in sperm, so they are transmitted only by females, through the egg, to all of their children.

Multifactorial inheritance: inheritance whereby a trait is determined by at least several genes in combination with environmental factors. Multifactorial traits are familial, but do not follow the Mendelian laws.

Mutation: a random, permanent change in the genetic material, often due to a mistake when the DNA copies itself before cell division.

Nucleotide base pairs: there are four nitrogenous bases in the DNA: guanine (G), cytosine (C), adenine (A), and thymine (T), that are paired—G with C and A with T. Each base is combined with a sugar and a phosphate group to form a nucleotide.

Penetrance: a gene that always causes a condition when present in a single dose is said to be dominant with complete penetrance. If it fails to cause the condition in some carriers, it is said to have incomplete, or reduced, penetrance. The penetrance of a dominant gene is the proportion of people who carry it and have the condition.

Proteins: molecules that constitute the bulk of the body tissues, e.g., myoglobin (muscle), keratin (hair, nails, teeth), collagen (cartilage, tendons, skin), and hemoglobin (red blood cells). They are made up of long chains of amino acids. The sequence of amino acids determines the structure, and so the function, of the protein.

Recessive: a recessive form of a gene (allele) is one that is expressed only when it is combined with another recessive like itself, and not in the presence of a dominant form.

Regression to the mean: a rule that states that for any multifactorial trait, such as height, the average value of the children will be halfway between the average of the parents and that of the population. So the offspring of tall parents, for example, will be on average shorter than their parents, but taller than the population average.

Sex chromosome: one of the pair of chromosomes, X and Y, that determine sex. A person with two X-chromosomes is a female; a person with an X and a Y is a male.

Sibs, siblings: brothers and sisters. Strictly speaking, a sibling is a little sib, but usage seems to favor this diminutive, rather than sib, the more correct form.

SNP: single nucleotide polymorphism. A difference between individuals in a single base pair. Most SNPs are harmless, but they are frequent (about one in every one thousand base pairs) and can be used to map the chromosomal location of a gene.

Syndrome: a characteristic association of several anomalies in the same individual, suggesting that they have the same cause—e.g., trisomy 21 or Down syndrome.

Trisomy 21: a condition where an extra chromosome 21 (three instead of two) causes a characteristic pattern of defects and minor anomalies. See Down syndrome.

Turner syndrome: see XO Turner syndrome.

Twin studies: A classic approach to the question of how much genes and environment contribute to the variation in a particular trait. It compares the similarity to one another, with respect to the trait, of pairs of monozygotic (MZ) and dizygotic (DZ) twins. MZ twins arise from the splitting of one egg, and are genetically identical. DZ pairs arise from the concurrent fertilization of two eggs, and are no more alike genetically than ordinary sibs. The more alike MZ pairs are than DZ pairs, with respect to the trait, the greater the genetic contribution—i.e., the higher the heritability.

XO Turner syndrome: a syndrome resulting from absence of one of the two X chromosomes as in a normal female.

Y chromosome: the sex chromosome that determines maleness. An XX person is female; an XY person is a male.

Further Reading

Here are some suggestions for those who would like to explore further the role of genes in their genealogy.

Books

There are a number of books that expand on the material in chapter one on how DNA is used to trace your ancestry. I'll mention but two of them:

Fitzpatrick, Colleen and Andrew Yelser. DNA and Genealogy. Rice Book Press, 2005.

Smolenyak, Megan and Ann Turner. *Trace your Roots with DNA*. Rodale, 2004.

There are many books on the practical details of tracing your family tree, searching birth and death records, obituaries, medical records, and the like, and also drawing your pedigree on your computer. A good one is

Shawker, Thomas H. *Unlocking your Genetic History*. Rutledge Press, 2004.

If you want to get into the details of human genetics, there are lots of good texts. Unfortunately, mine are out of print. Many of them are oriented to medical students, but nevertheless quite understandable to the layperson. For example:

Cummings, Michael. *Human Heredity, Principles and Issues.* Brooks/Cole Publishing, 2003.

Nussbaum, Robert, Roderick McInnes, and Huntington Willard. *Thompson and Thompson, Genetics in Medicine.* Saunders, 2004.

Some are more directly aimed at laypersons. For example:

Lewis, Ricki. *Human Genetics: Concepts and Applications.* McGraw-Hill, 2005.

Online

There is a bewildering array of information sources on the Web, of varying degrees of reliability. Pay attention to the sources. If they are university Web sites or prestigious sources such as NIH, they are likely to be reliable. Other sources should be regarded with a raised eyebrow. They may be OK, but they may *not* be. Among the reliable sources are:

Online Mendelian Inheritance in Man (OMIM), an online version of McKusick's Catalog of Mendelian Inheritance in Man. It is a historical record of the research on every known condition with a genetic basis. For a layperson, or even a professional, the voluminous array of information on many conditions may be formidable, but if you are willing to wade through a lot of material, you can find out what is known about the genetic basis of any human condition. Google OMIM. You can also check the library for the four-volume printed version.

PubMed, www.ncbi.nlm.nih.gov/entrez, a service of the United States National Library of Medicine includes over sixteen million references for biomedical articles back to the 1950's. Simply type in the condition you want and genetics, and it will list all the articles on that subject. Type in 1996 to 2006 to get recent references and keep the list down to a reasonable number.

The Centre for Genetics Education, http://www.genetics.com.au/, an Australian service dedicated to providing current and relevant genetics information to individuals and family members affected by genetic conditions. It provides information on genetics and on the genetics of specific conditions.

A Revolution in Progress: Human Genetics and Medical Research, http://www.history.nih.gov/exhibits/genetics/, an NIH production that is a nice layperson's introduction to basic genetics and its modern impact.

Explore and enjoy.

About the Author

Clarke Fraser was born in 1920, and spent much of his childhood in Jamaica, but his cultural roots were in Nova Scotia. He gained a BSc at Acadia University in Nova Scotia in 1940, and a PhD in Genetics from McGill University, Montreal, in 1943. After three years in the Royal Canadian Air Force, he went back to McGill and earned his MD degree in 1950, thus becoming Canada's first Medical Geneticist.

For the next forty-nine years he busied himself at McGill, with teaching, research, and developing the principles of genetic counseling at the Clinical Genetics Unit—which he started—at The Montreal Children's Hospital.

Fraser did pioneering research in three areas, the genetics of human disorders, genetic counseling, and teratology (the experimental production of birth defects (in mice)), being the first to bring genetics into this new field He also trained many graduate and post-doctoral students, who have gone on to productive careers in medical genetics or teratology in various parts of the world.

Clarke Fraser wrote some three hundred papers on human genetics and teratology, co-edited a four-volume Handbook of Teratology, and co-authored two textbooks on Human and Medical Genetics. He is a Fellow of the Royal Society of Canada, was appointed an Officer of the Order of Canada in 1985, and received a number of awards, including the Blackader Award of the Canadian Medical Association (1968), the Allen award (1978), and the Award of Excellence in Education (2000) from the American Society of Human Genetics. He also received the Wilder Penfield Prix de Quebec (1999), as well as three honorary degrees, from Acadia (1967), New York at Potsdam (1995), and Dalhousie University (2003).

Clarke served on a number of national and international committees, including the Canadian MRC Committee on Genetics, the NIH Genetics Study Section, and the WHO Expert Advisory Committee on Human Genetics. He was President of the American Society of Human Genetics, the Teratology Society, and the Canadian College of Medical Geneticists. From 1990 to 1993 he served as head of the working group on genetics and prenatal diagnosis of the Canadian Royal Commission on New Reproductive Technologies.

In 1999, Clarke Fraser and his wife, Dr Marilyn Preus, retired to his ancestral home in Nova Scotia, but he maintains his Emeritus Professorship at McGill, and is still writing papers—and this book.

Index

978-0-595-39686-3
0-595-39686-0

Printed in the United States
59440LVS00005B/522